EARLY PARENTHOOD
AND COMING OF
AGE IN THE 1990s

D1441236

EARLY PARENTHOOD AND COMING OF AGE IN THE 1990s

edited by
MARGARET K. ROSENHEIM
and MARK F. TESTA

RUTGERS UNIVERSITY PRESS

NEW BRUNSWICK, NEW JERSEY

Library of Congress Cataloging-in-Publication Data

Early parenthood and coming of age in the 1990s / edited by Margaret
K. Rosenheim and Mark F. Testa.
    p. cm.
    Includes bibliographical references and index.
    ISBN 0-8135-1815-6 (cloth)—ISBN 0-8135-1816-4 (pbk.)
    1. Teenage parents—United States. 2. Adulthood—United States.
3. Teenagers—United States—Economic conditions. 4. Teenage
pregnancy—United States—Prevention. 5. Teenage parents—
Government policy—United States. I. Rosenheim, Margaret K.
(Margaret Keeney), 1926– . II. Testa, Mark.
HQ759.64.E27 1992
306.85'6—dc20   91-40325
                                                                        CIP

British Cataloging-in-Publication information available

Contents

Figures

Tables

Preface

Early Parenthood and Coming of Age in the 1990s is the first publication to result from a project on The Public World of Childhood. This phrase, The Public World of Childhood, is meant to capture what we see as noteworthy features of bringing up children and youth in contemporary American society. It is intended to direct attention to the fact that, over the years from birth to majority, young people spend a vast amount of time outside the home and, whether within or without it, beyond the immediate direction of parents or other responsible surrogates. What children and adolescents actually do under these circumstances is a matter of great concern to most parents. It is also, at least intermittently, a matter of concern to the public at large.

The teen years are a particularly important focus of public concern. As rapidly maturing human beings, adolescents enjoy increasing freedom in their daily affairs. Enticements to test out the limits of freedom abound, as do the possibilities for long-lasting harm. Sexual exploration is one avenue of conduct that may well affect the course of a teenager's life. An example of life-altering consequence is conduct that results in early pregnancy or—even more dramatically—in early parenthood.

In considering the problems identified with pregnancy and parenthood at an early age, we have sought to use the perspectives of a Public World of Childhood. We place the discussion of early parenthood against the backdrop of youth's extending economic and social dependency, a phenomenon characteristic of the industrialized nations of the world. We also take note of trends affecting family oversight and the supplementation, or replacement, of familial responsibility with informal mechanisms, such as the peer group, and formal institutions, such as schools, welfare offices, and juvenile courts. We draw on the insights of scholars and public leaders from different areas of specialization in order to achieve a multifaceted view of the topic at hand.

We are appreciative of the efforts of many people who have helped us discharge the task we envisioned.

We wish to make grateful acknowledgment of financial support from The Joyce Foundation, as well as the thoughtful encouragement of the foundation's president, Craig Kennedy. We are appreciative of the able assistance of the foundation's program associates who saw to our grant: Adam Clement, Marta White, and Zaverie Moore.

Early on, even before we sought out foundation support, we were pleased to receive encouragement from former dean Harold Richman for our individual efforts, which came to fruition in the work of The Public World of Childhood. We also feel special gratitude for the confidence and support, during the years of the project's operation, of two other deans of the School of Social Service Administration at the University of Chicago—Laurence Lynn and Jeanne Marsh.

We are fortunate to have had an interdisciplinary group of faculty colleagues whose generous advice is always forthcoming. We thank them all for their ideas, criticism, and insight, and wish to extend special acknowledgment to Norval Morris, Mary Becker, Kirsten Grønbjerg, William Pollak, Marta Tienda, Jon Conte, and Michael Sosin for their participation. We appreciate especially many conversations with Arthur Kohrman and Franklin Zimring, each of whom helped us shape the conception of The Public World of Childhood and offered astute insights on the topic of early parenthood. Jacqueline Forrest of the Alan Guttmacher Institute enriched our understanding of comparative international trends. We are also grateful to Jennifer Knauss of the Illinois Caucus on Teenage Pregnancy for helping us convene groups of advocates and community leaders, whose articulate and thoughtful comments proved so valuable to our reflections.

Our staff of project directors, research assistants, and support personnel have made possible the many undertakings that have enabled our plans and investigations to achieve fruition in this volume. We thank Anne Wells for the important contributions she made as the first project director of The Public World of Childhood. We appreciate the intellect, ingenuity, energy, and patience demonstrated by the many research assistants who have worked on this project: Ann Raney, Joy Workman, Ki Whan Kim, Betse Thielman, Sandra Keifert, Jayesh Shah, Moon-kie Jung, and Paul Custer. The work of all these people was also supported by the school's typists and Keith Madderom and Beverly Mason of the administrative staff of the School of Social Service Administration. Finally, we wish to extend our deep appreciation to Sandy Dixon, project director of The Public World of Childhood, for her enormous contributions and dedicated leadership in bringing this work to successful completion.

Margaret K. Rosenheim
Mark F. Testa
Chicago, December 1991

EARLY PARENTHOOD
AND COMING OF
AGE IN THE 1990s

MARK F. TESTA

Introduction

The problem of teenage parenthood is being reconsidered. Teenage parenthood was identified in the 1970s as being chiefly a public health concern; the prognosis was that its levels would gradually decline as adolescents' sexual education and access to contraceptives and abortion improved. However, although teen birthrates in the United States are lower by almost 50 percent than in the 1950s, there have been no significant reductions in either teenage pregnancy or childbearing rates since the mid-1970s. Between 1986 and 1989, teen birthrates increased 15 percent to their highest level in fifteen years (National Center for Health Statistics 1991). This lack of progress, despite more than a decade and a half of public and private support for services and research, plus startling new evidence about the health and developmental consequences of early parenthood, are prompting a rethinking of public policies toward prevention of teenage pregnancy and support for adolescent parents in the 1990s (Luker 1991).

To what extent is teenage pregnancy simply the accidental result of unprotected sexual intercourse? Would postponing childbearing beyond the teenage years substantially improve infant survival rates? How consequential is early parenthood for the future social and economic well-being of parents and children? These are just some of the questions that seemed answered a few years ago but are now being asked again. More often than not, the answers that the latest research is providing appear to contradict many of once-accepted responses. Some of the revisions gaining currency follow. (1) A substantial portion of teenage pregnancy is not accidental but rather the conscious choice of a stratum of disadvantaged adolescents who perceive little gain from delaying parenthood (Dash 1989). (2) Early pregnancy is not inherently detrimental to infant survival but is correlated with socioeconomic disadvantages that impair parental and child health regardless of maternal age (Geronimus 1987). (3) Early motherhood does not invariably produce educational failure and economic privation but does often result in socioeconomic achievements that are no worse than those of women in similar circumstances who postpone parenthood (Upchurch and McCarthy 1990).

Although this latest evidence could be construed as repudiating all earlier understanding of the problem, the newer results are better interpreted as a diversification of our knowledge. Accidental pregnancies undeniably account for a large portion of teenage pregnancy, as indicated by the fact that some 40 percent of pregnant teens each year elect to have abortions. Yet our knowledge about those who carry their pregnancies to term is less firm. Also, early childbearing is statistically associated with ill health for both mother and infant, but medical authorities disagree about the biological importance of early maternal age, particularly when the adolescent is over fifteen. Likewise, women who begin having children before completing the normative transitions of finishing school, entering the work force, or marrying run a higher risk of long-term poverty and welfare dependency. But this higher risk does not obviate the chance that, with appropriate assistance and support, many parents can find an acceptable route to self-sufficient adulthood.

The debate generated by the recent findings on early parenthood has led to greater acknowledgment of the need to build into both the prevention of teenage pregnancy and the support of adolescent parents more awareness of the diversity of early parenthood across social and cultural contexts. Research shows that the medical risks, social sanctions, and forms of support that a teen can expect if she becomes pregnant vary with her age, race, and class. Although we speak of teenage parenthood as if the problem were generic, it takes on very different meaning and significance depending on whether the subject is a minor under fifteen or a teenage adult over eighteen. Similarly, one cannot assume that all teenagers have identical stakes in postponing parenthood. The fact that adolescent motherhood occurs disproportionately among minority and socioeconomically disadvantaged youth suggests that the prevention of early pregnancy may not just be a matter of instructing adolescents about contraceptives, family planning, and life options. It may require major initiatives to deal with the underlying socioeconomic and cultural conditions that encourage the high levels of early childbearing among minority and lower-class youth in this country.

The purpose of this volume is to contribute to an understanding of the diversity of early parenthood by considering the different social and cultural contexts in which teenage childbearing occurs. The essays are cross-disciplinary and represent the best recent national and international scholarship on early parenthood. They draw on theoretical developments and empirical findings from psychology, medicine, social work, history, sociology, and law. By considering how the contexts of early parenthood have changed historically, compare cross-nationally, and differ by age, race, and class in the United States, the essays try to clarify the nature of the contemporary problem of teenage parenthood and to sharpen the focus of policies aimed at preventing teenage pregnancy and supporting adolescent parents and their children.

Early Parenthood and the Transition to Adulthood

A common theme of these essays is that the contemporary problem of teenage parenthood needs to be understood within the larger institutional context of the extended social and economic dependency of all youth in modern society. Few persons under twenty years old today are in the economic position of the prior two generations to marry and to start a family shortly after graduating from high school. The industrial economy that once supported large numbers of youth in well-paying manual and unskilled jobs has shrunk and given way to a service economy that pays the minimum wage or requires at least a college diploma or advanced training for better-paid employment. The decline in manufacturing jobs, along with the rise in educational requirements for full economic participation, has rendered almost obsolete (except for part-time work) the economic function of an entire stratum of youth under age twenty. As a consequence, the transition from adolescent dependence to economic independence typically lasts well past the teenage years into most young persons' middle or late twenties.

The extension of adolescent dependency into the third decade of life requires young people to follow a lengthened social timetable for when they complete their education, school, enter the labor force, marry, and become parents. On the one hand, there is evidence that increasing numbers of youth are adapting to the upward revision of age-graded norms, as indicated, for example, by later median ages at school completion, marriage, and parenthood. On the other, there is evidence that the pace of adaptation is lagging, especially among low-income and minority youth, as indicated by rising levels of out-of-wedlock births, single-parent families, and long-term welfare dependency. Increasingly, deviance from a lengthened social timetable of adolescent development via early pregnancy and parenthood raises the incidence of single parenthood and family poverty because of the shrinking social and economic opportunities for youth to achieve self-sufficiency through employment and marriage. The resulting paradox is that although teenage birthrates have plummeted from the levels of three decades ago, early parenthood continues to intensify as a social problem.

An Epidemic of Teenage Pregnancy?

When teenage pregnancy and parenthood first became national concerns in the late 1970s, the prevailing public health view of pregnancy prevention led easily to the characterization of the problem as an "epidemic." Although the linkage to the prevention of communicable diseases did attract public attention, the misleading impression was that teenage pregnancy and parenthood were rapidly on the rise in the United States. On the contrary, teenage pregnancy rates were no higher in the 1970s than in the 1950s. Furthermore, teenage childbearing rates were down substantially from 90 births per 1,000 girls aged 15–19 in the 1950s to somewhat more than 50 births per 1,000 girls aged 15–19 in the 1970s. In both absolute and proportionate terms, there were more babies born to adolescents before the so-called epidemic of teenage pregnancy than after. Why, then, did the matter gain national attention only in the late 1970s?

Maris Vinovskis addresses this question in his essay "Historical Perspectives on Adolescent Pregnancy." Despite the higher numbers, he observes, teenage parenthood was not widely perceived as a social problem in the 1950s. This was because early childbearing occurred almost invariably within the confines of marriage. As recently as 1960, about 85 percent of births to mothers under twenty occurred after marriage. Even among the very youngest of mothers, aged fourteen or younger, about 30 percent of births were to married girls (National Center for Health Statistics 1962). Although many of the marriages were hastily arranged to cover up a premarital pregnancy, it is estimated that over one-half of the first children borne by teenagers during the 1950s were conceived after the couple's wedding (O'Connell and Rogers 1984). Although hardly encouraged, teenage marriage and motherhood were tolerated because they accelerated only slightly women's normal developmental life course and carried only moderate opportunity costs. Women's expected careers still centered on marriage and motherhood.

All of this began to change in the 1960s. Feminist ideology and the lowering of gender barriers to occupational achievement gradually opened alternative career paths for women. This led, in turn, to higher levels of female enrollment in college and to later marriage. The proportion of U.S. women aged eighteen to nineteen years enrolled in college grew from 23 percent in 1955 to 44 percent in 1989 (U.S. Bureau of the Census 1991a). During the same period, 18–19-year-old women who had ever married dropped from 32 percent to under 10 percent. This shift in female roles from teen brides to college students had an inhibiting effect on teen fertility levels: They fell from a high of 96 births per 1,000 women aged 15–19 in 1957 to a low of somewhat fewer than 51 births per 1,000 in 1986 (National Center for Health Statistics 1990). Most of the decline occurred among women eighteen to nineteen years old.

The Deregulation of Premarital Sexual Relations

The postponement of school completion, marriage, and parenthood extended the normal adolescent life course for youth growing up in the 1970s beyond their teenage years into their twenties. One developmental milestone that was reached at a younger age, however, was the initiation of sexual activity. The proportion of women aged fifteen to nineteen who reported having sexual intercourse rose from an estimated 33 percent in 1970 to 46 percent in the early 1980s (Hofferth and Hayes 1987). The latest survey figures indicate that over half (53 percent) of teenage females have had sexual intercourse (Forrest and Singh 1990).

The rise in teenage sexual activity during this period was not an isolated phenomenon; it was related to the general easing of public attitudes against premarital sexual relations. Opinion polls of the American population show that the proportion of women who answered it is "not wrong at all" if a man and a woman have sexual relations before marriage increased from 19 percent in 1972 to 34 percent in 1988. Among men, the increase was from 34 to 46 percent (Niemi et al. 1988). As long as public opinion considered premarital sexual relations as immoral, families and communities could rely on marital norms to regulate adolescent sexual activity through the government's enforcing age limits on marriage and society's discouraging marriage until economic independence was a realistic possibility. But as public tolerance for premarital sexual relations increased and the predictable age at marriage extended past twenty, the force of the argument "wait until you are married" began to lose much of its normative significance to teenagers. What followed was an unprecedented rise in premarital pregnancies and out-of-wedlock births to teens.

Between 1960 and 1989, the number of births to unmarried girls aged between fifteen and nineteen years increased from 87,000 to 337,000. Expressed as a rate per 1,000 unmarried women, the rise in nonmarital childbearing was significant—from 15 births per 1,000 women in 1960 to 41 births per 1,000 women in 1989. As a ratio of nonmarital to total births, the rise was truly phenomenal. In 1960, about 15 percent of all births to teenagers were to unmarried mothers. A decade later, it had doubled to 30 percent; by 1985, it had doubled again to nearly 60 percent. As of 1989, 67 percent of teenage mothers were unwed when they gave birth. Out-of-wedlock childbearing became the modal experience of teenage parents during the 1980s.

The prevention of premarital pregnancy among teenagers became an explicit target of public intervention with the 1975 revisions of the federal Title X Family Planning Services and Research Act. The following year, the Alan Guttmacher Institute issued its landmark report, *11 Million Teenagers: What Can Be Done about the Epidemic of Adolescent Pregnancies in the United States* (1976). The report's framing the problem in terms of chronological age rather than marital status was intended to communicate the opinion that adolescent pregnancy was harmful to the well-being of young women whether the birth occurred in or outside of marriage. It also helped to distance the discussion from the controversy generated by the 1965 appearance of Moynihan's *Negro Family: The Case for National Action*. This government report, written by then Assistant Secretary of Labor Daniel Patrick Moynihan, identified out-of-wedlock childbearing as one of the chief impediments to blacks' achieving economic parity with whites. Family planning advocates were able to maintain the necessary political coalition that supported public action by discouraging early parenthood rather than extramarital parenthood. Chronological age still is one of the few bases of ascriptive differentiation that continue to legitimate subordinate status at a time when most others have been discarded as politically unworkable.

The Age Grading of Sexual and Reproductive Behavior

All modern societies rely to some extent on age grading to regulate human behavior. Social scientists use the term to refer to society's use of chronological age as a basis for assigning roles and defining statuses in the allocation of permissions, rights, and obligations. In the United States, we establish varying age restrictions on when adolescents can leave school, obtain employment, marry, consume alcoholic beverages, and participate in the political process. Parents use age-graded norms as reference points for judging whether their children are advanced or behind in their development and whether adolescents are precocious or immature in their behavior. Considered as a form of age grading, prevention of teenage parenthood can be subsumed under the broader set of adjustment problems that arise whenever a society undertakes to revise its age-graded norms upward to limit youth's access to adult economic, social, and political roles and privileges. At the turn of the century, laws on compulsory education, child labor, and juvenile delinquency institutionalized a new stage of adolescent dependency in the life cycle by limiting youth's autonomy and participation in adult life. Modern policies to prevent teenage pregnancy attempt to accomplish the same by discouraging early sex and opposing premature transitions to parenthood.

The affinity between teenage pregnancy and other forms of juvenile deviance is explored in Anne Petersen and Lisa Crockett's chapter "Adolescent Sexuality, Pregnancy, and Child Bearing: Developmental Perspectives." Much of what we label as problem behavior among juveniles arises from their failure to abide by rules that prohibit or discourage them from engaging precociously in acts that are permissible for adults. These include drinking alcohol, staying out late (violating curfew), leaving home (running away), and being absent from school without excuse (being truant). Sexual activity is also in this category of behavior, even though the age boundaries are less plainly drawn in law.

A good deal of research on the correlates and antecedents of early sexual activity, pregnancy, and parenthood finds a close association between them and other forms of juvenile deviance, such as smoking, absence from school, drinking alcohol, and mild delinquency (Jessor and Jessor 1975; Hogan 1984; Abrahamse et al. 1988). Explanations for the association range from juveniles' conformity to peer influences that encourage deviant or rebellious behavior to their psychological readiness to engage in adult behaviors—what the Jessors call "transition proneness." Related to this idea is Petersen and Crockett's finding in their study of rural adolescents that girls who have engaged in coitus expected to make earlier transitions to work, marriage, and parenthood than did girls who were not yet sexually active. Petersen and Crockett also report that early sexual activity is negatively related to high educational aspirations, a finding that agrees with those of other studies (Abrahamse et al. 1988). Taken together, these results support the classic formulation on juvenile deviance that hypothesizes that readiness to comply with a set of age-graded norms varies with young people's assessments of how much their future life chances depend on their present conformity to or divergence from these norms.

Class and Race

Delaying marriage, completing college studies, and postponing parenthood are society's prescriptions for achieving positions of middle-class earnings, power, and prestige. Lower-class and minority youth are less likely to postpone parenthood than upper-class and nonminority youth. The basic pattern can be illustrated with data from a 1980–1982 panel study of a nationally representative sample of high school sophomores.[1] By their senior year (or what would have been if all had remained in school) an estimated 4.5 percent of never-married, childless sophomore girls had become mothers. Girls in the lowest socioeconomic quartile were four times more likely to have a child than girls in the highest socioeconomic quartile, regardless of race. Black girls were also three times more likely to have a child than non-Hispanic white girls, regardless of socioeconomic status. If the comparisons were limited to unmarried mothers, the racial differentials would be even greater.

Research has long shown that lower-class and minority youth become sexually active younger, have higher rates of teen pregnancy, and are more likely to have a child than upper-class and nonminority youth. What is less well known is that rates of black teenage unwed childbearing, unlike white rates, declined for much of the last two decades—from 98 births per 1,000 unmarried teenagers in the early 1970s to 86 births per 1,000 unmarried teenagers in the early 1980s.[2] But in 1985, the trend abruptly reversed.

Figure I.1 illustrates the dramatic turnaround in unwed childbearing among black adolescents. As of 1989, the birthrate among black unwed teens aged 18 to 19 years had climbed past its 1970 level to 147 births per 1,000 unmarried teenagers and among black teens aged 15 to 17 years to

FIGURE I.1

Nonmarital Fertility Rates, by Race and Age, United States, 1970–1989

RATE PER 1,000 UNMARRIED WOMEN

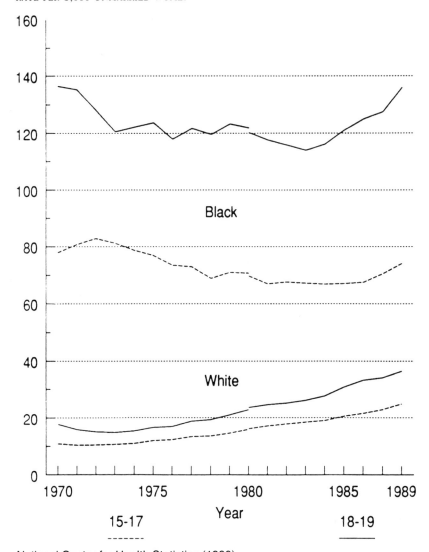

National Center for Health Statistics (1990).

its 1974 level of 79 births per 1,000 unmarried teenagers. Without more recent data on contraceptive use and abortion, it is difficult to sort out the reasons for the sharp upturn in black teen birthrates. Although it may be that black unwed childbearing rates will decline again in the 1990s, there is reason to suspect that the incentives for lower-class and minority adolescents to conform to a social timetable for prolonged transition to adulthood are weakening. Given the diminished importance of marriage as a normative prerequisite to childbearing, the possibility must be seriously entertained that the recent rise in levels of teenage childbearing is not simply the chance result of unprotected sexual intercourse but may reflect teenagers' decisions to deviate from society's age-graded pathway to adulthood (Hogan and Astone 1986).

In her chapter "Early Childbearing Patterns among African Americans: A Socio-historical Perspective," Donna Franklin traces the changing social and cultural contexts of black out-of-wedlock childbearing from the outlawing of marriage under the institution of American slavery to the rising public concern over the concentration of single-parent families in "underclass" ghettos and public housing high-rises. She notes that, although most scholarly research has tended to interpret black unwed childbearing as part of a "tangle of pathology" (Clark 1967) or a manifestation of a "culture of poverty" (Lewis 1961), other research has drawn attention to its adaptive features for women and children whose situation was not necessarily improved through delaying childbirth. This other view raises the possibility that continuing high levels of black teenage parenthood may not reflect a rejection of middle-class norms of achievement but rather adolescents' conscious choice of an alternative life course (Hamburg 1986; Geronimus 1987; Burton 1990).

Alternative Life Course

Such a hypothesis is presented in Beatrix Hamburg and Sandra Dixon's chapter "Adolescent Pregnancy and Parenthood." They draw on social surveys and ethnographic research in suggesting that early childbearing may be functional for low-income, black adolescents in ways that are not the same for middle-class, white adolescents. In fact, they argue, low-income, black adolescents may perceive that having children is preferable to waiting. If one considers the fact that health and marriage prospects, unlike those for white women, do not improve substantially when black women enter their twenties, it may make sense for a low-income, black adolescent to begin her childbearing when she is a teenager so that she can draw on public aid and the support of parents and grandparents for child care while she completes her schooling. During her late teens, she can use the time to expand and solidify her extended kin network in preparation for establishing her own household. By the time she is ready to enter the work force, her children will be old enough to go to grade school and to help around the house. With childbearing completed before age twenty, she is able to participate fully in the labor force without the time-out for childbirth and the high costs of infant care associated with delayed childbearing.

This is, of course, a startling and somewhat heretical proposition. In order to grasp the underlying logic, it is important to have some understanding of the inner-city environment in which many low-income, black adolescents are growing up in the United States. Jewelle Taylor Gibbs presents a disturbing picture of urban ghetto life in her "Social Context of Teenage Pregnancy and Parenting in the Black Community: Implications for Public Policy." She draws attention to the problematic circumstances of young black males in the inner city who, at ages twenty to twenty-four, are most likely to father the children of teenage women. She cites numbing statistics on the high levels of high school drop-outs, joblessness, delinquency, crime, incarceration, drug use, and murder. Considered separately, any one of these gives cause for concern; together, they signify a crisis of staggering magnitude.

The cumulative effect of these multiple hazards of ghetto life has been to deplete the available pool of employable and responsible marital partners for black women in their prime years of family formation. One adaptation to the shortage of marriageable men has been the detachment of sexual relations, childbearing, and parenthood from the institution of marriage. Few black women in inner-city neighborhoods marry before having children, and the number who remain unmarried during their children's early formative years has grown in recent decades. The proportion of black children living in mother-only families has risen 70 percent since 1970 from 30 to 51 percent in 1989, while the subset living with parents who have never married has risen an astounding 575 percent from 4 to 27 percent (U.S. Bureau of the Census 1990). Gibbs observes that the concentration of mother-only families in public highrises and ghetto communities leads to a special kind of social isolation that enables residents to adjust to their disadvantages by accepting, if not condoning, nonmarital unions and the pervasive absence of fathers from homes. Their social isolation reinforces ghetto-specific behaviors and norms that, while adaptive to inner-city contingencies, are at sharp variance with the norms and values of the wider society.

Adolescent Welfare Dependency

Most popular discussions of adolescent family life in the ghetto emphasize the deviant, disorderly, and destructive aspects of out-of-wedlock, teenage childbearing. The alternative life-course perspective lends some balance to this by drawing attention to the functional adaptations that black families have been able to make to shield their daughters from experiencing to the full the negative consequences usually associated with early childbearing in the United States. Mark Testa examines the modal responses of parents and daughters to early childbirth in a sample of adolescent welfare mothers in his "Racial and Ethnic Variation in the Early Life Course of Adolescent Welfare Mothers." He finds that black girls were more likely to remain in their parental home after childbirth, continue in school, and delay marriage than white and Hispanic girls, who were more likely to follow the traditional route of leaving home, dropping out of school, and, when the opportunity arose, marrying. Although the latter set of responses was associated with shorter durations of welfare receipt, the former was associated with higher educational attainment. A longer period of follow-up will be necessary to determine whether the alternative life course results in the same or higher levels of future self-sufficiency as those attained by adolescent mothers who follow the more traditional route of school drop-out, departure from the home, and early marriage.

The point of these findings is not to glorify or romanticize the alternative life course. It is even unclear the extent to which the pattern commands affirmative allegiance in poor communities as a design for living. For the moment, the alternative life course is best regarded as a "semi-institutionalized" response to the limited opportunities to which urban black families have been able to adapt. By drawing on their ethnic heritage and cultural resources to develop coping mechanisms and informal systems of mutual support, they lower the long-term "opportunity costs" of their daughters' becoming single teenage parents. Recent evidence shows that black women do not gain as much from delaying childbearing as white women do in infant health, educational attainment, and income (Geronimus 1987; Lundberg and Plotnick 1989). Although such findings appear to support the viability of the alternative life course, to evaluate fully the effects of this situational adaptation, prospective longitudinal studies are needed that follow teenage parents from adolescence through young adulthood into middle age and assess the well-being of both parents and children.

One of the classic longitudinal studies of teenage parenthood is the Baltimore study of 400 teenage mothers who received prenatal care at the city's Sinai Hospital. Frank Furstenberg, Mary Elizabeth Hughes, and Jeanne Brooks-Gunn pick up the story of these young women and their children in "The Next Generation: The Children of Teenage Mothers Grow Up." Furstenberg and his associates have been documenting the changes in the lives of these women and their children in a number of landmark investigations of the long-term consequences of teenage childbearing. Twenty years separates the latest round of interviews conducted in 1987 from the original ones done between 1966 and 1968. Their follow-ups show that many of the teenage mothers were able to complete high school, find employment, and move off welfare, confirming the diversity of outcomes for adolescent mothers in later life. The same holds true for the majority of their children who, despite registering higher levels of juvenile deviance than a sample of youth whose mothers had delayed childbearing, were making reasonable progress toward independent adulthood. Furstenberg, Hughes, and Brooks-Gunn rightly point out that this diversity of outcomes belies the overly deterministic view of the consequences of growing up poor in the household of a teenage parent. Given their disadvantages, it is rather extraordinary that so many children were able to make their way into the mainstream. The question left open is whether, with better support and assistance, an even larger percentage of these youth would have been able to overcome the disadvantages of their childhood environments.

Pregnancy Prevention and Family Support

The developmental conditions of adolescence in the 1990s—the extension of the social and economic dependency of youth, the loss of the regulatory force of norms against premarital sex, and the semi-institutionalization of an alternative life course among early childbearers—pose formidable challenges to the prevention of teenage pregnancy and to adolescent family support. Some argue that abstinence is the best solution. Yet the marginal results of the "just say no" campaign of the 1980s to promote premarital continence suggest that current levels of adolescent sexual activity are unlikely to fall, the AIDS peril notwithstanding. Others promote sex education and easier access to contraceptives and abortion. While social surveys show that contraceptive practice among adolescents has improved, especially in the use of condoms (Mosher 1990), the rise in birthrates among the unwed leaves doubts as to whether the incentives for delayed childbirth, particularly among lower-class and minority youth, are sufficient to reverse current trends. Others see the prevention of damage to children as the more critical objective. If out-of-wedlock birthrates continue to rise, the support of mother-only families will certainly need to assume a higher budgetary priority to safeguard the welfare of early parents and their children. The concern, however, is that improved support will lessen the incentives to delay parenthood in the first place.

Efforts to arrive at a more consistent policy of teenage pregnancy prevention and adolescent family support were stalemated in the 1980s as political forces clashed over whether to expand external controls over adolescent sexual and reproductive behavior by mandating parental involvement in minors' obtaining contraceptives and abortions or to encourage internal controls by promoting sex education in the schools and guaranteeing privacy of access to family planning services. Although the controversy is far from finished, the backers of greater parental involvement scored important victories in drawing distinctions between the permissions, rights, and obligations of minor parents and teenage adult parents over seventeen. These distinctions eventually found their way into the 1988 Family Support Act, which imposes special restrictions on minor parents' rights to receive public assistance. It is uncertain how much headway the push to contract further the autonomy of minors in sexual and reproductive decision making is likely to gain in the 1990s, but, as Franklin Zimring warns in "The Jurisprudence of Teenage Pregnancy," a half-century's experience with prevention of juvenile delinquency indicates that paternalistic and coercive interventions to enforce age-graded norms often do not produce results worth the price of the anguish they inflict.

International Comparisons

The social and cultural conditions under which paternalistic policies are likely to succeed are changing in traditional societies as well as modern ones. Korea is a nation that ranks much lower than the United States in rates of teenage pregnancy and parenthood. The major reason, as explained by Kyu-taik Sung in his "Teenage Pregnancy and Premarital Childbirth in Korea: Issues and Concerns," is Korean society's reluctance to recognize and accept sexual relations outside of marriage. Arranged marriages are still quite common, and most young people report a preference for marriages where parents consent to the selection of the spouse-to-be. The ability of Korean traditions to withstand the pressures of modern change remains an open question. But Sung already senses that Korean society will eventually need to take greater cognizance of the problem of teenage pregnancy as rates of cohabitation and premarital sexual relations rise with the urbanization of the population. He argues that coming to terms with these developments will require wider acknowledgment of the risks of premarital sexual relations and greater emphasis on more effective contraception by young people.

Swedish social customs have long since passed the stage when sexual relations and childbearing were sanctioned only within marriage. Yet Sweden also ranks much lower than the United States in rates of teenage pregnancy and parenthood despite its having one of the world's most generous family welfare policies. In her "Early Phases of Family Formation in Contemporary Sweden," Britta Hoem attributes these lower rates to the young person's desires to complete his or her education, settle into an occupation, and enjoy his or her leisure time without being encumbered by the responsibilities of early parenthood. The successful adaptation of most Swedish youth to the norms of delayed parenthood, in spite of permissive sexual attitudes and generous support for single-parent families, suggests that the trade-offs between teenage pregnancy prevention and adolescent family support may not be as stark as they are often argued. The more critical factor appears to be how much young people feel that they have a stake in complying with a prolonged social timetable of human development. Swedish social policy guarantees free college education, aims at full employment, and entitles families to children's allowances and generous parental leave benefits. There is little gain in negotiating an alternative life course to adulthood in Sweden.

Lessons for the 1990s

The lessons in this volume of essays will likely be hard ones for some readers to accept. The data show that the contemporary problem of teenage parenthood cannot be understood simply as numerical, of rising numbers of teenagers having children. Teenage birthrates are still lower today than they were thirty years ago in spite of the recent upturn. Improved sex education and access to contraceptives and abortions are essential to effective pregnancy prevention and birth control, but only if pregnancies are unintended. Neither can the problem be blamed on generous welfare policies rewarding young unmarried women for having babies. The rate of out-of-wedlock childbearing among black adolescents was declining for most of the previous two decades. It was only after federal welfare programs were slashed in the mid-1980s and the median family income of black teen mothers had fallen to almost one-half its real dollar amount in the late 1970s (Duncan and Hoffman 1991) that we see adolescent birthrates rising among blacks. Countries with far more generous family welfare policies, such as Sweden, France, and Canada, have much lower levels of teenage pregnancy and parenthood than the United States (Jones et al. 1986).

The contemporary problem of teenage parenthood, as this volume attests, is the result of changing social context. The socially prescribed route to middle-class achievement takes longer today and requires more years of educational preparation before young people are able to attain the economic wherewithal to marry and to raise a family. The data show that adolescents from more advantaged classes or from nations that attempt to equalize the advantages are more likely to comply with the lengthened social timetable than those from more disadvantaged classes or from nations that tolerate greater social inequalities. So long as chances for middle-class achievement are unequally distributed, less advantaged youth will tend to deviate from the prescribed route or seek alternative ones that depart from the mainstream. The critical policy issue for the 1990s is the extent to which American society will seek to raise the level of compliance by evening out young people's stakes in delaying their transition to parenthood.

NOTES

1. These data were made available by the Data Archive on Adolescent Pregnancy Prevention, Sociometrics Corporation, Palo Alto, California. The data set entitled *1980–1982 U.S. National Study of High School and Beyond, Selected Variables: A Longitudinal Study of Female Sophomores* was prepared by Peter Morrison, Linda Waite, and Allan Abrahamse of the Rand Corporation, Santa Monica, California.

2. The rise in the out-of-wedlock birthrates among white teenagers reflects mainly the growth in premarital sexual activity.

BEATRIX A. HAMBURG and SANDRA LEE DIXON

1 Adolescent Pregnancy and Parenthood

Progress in preventing teenage pregnancy and childbearing has been slow and uneven in the United States, although the number and variety of public and private programs aimed at this goal have grown since 1980 (Hayes 1987; Henshaw et al. 1989). At each step toward becoming an adolescent mother—from the choice of delaying or initiating sex to the choice of aborting or carrying a pregnancy to term—reductions in the risk of early parenthood have shown little uniform change over time and few consistent patterns across social groups. This lack of uniformity and consistency, appraised with attention to ethnographic and demographic studies of adolescent sexuality, contributes to the recognition that interventions ought to be targeted to "subsets of adolescent mothers" (see Hamburg 1986). While one would not want to go off in all directions mounting interventions, the available evidence suggests that a uniform approach toward reducing adolescent pregnancy is neither desirable nor feasible.

The kind of intervention that can be expected to assist young people at risk of early parenthood depends on the type of response that communities, families, and the young people themselves make to the prospect of becoming parents in the teenage years. These responses include adoption or abortion to relinquish parenthood, early marriage to legitimate parenthood, and assistance from public and family sources to support single parenthood. We do not propose that these are definitive or exhaustive categorizations, but we have found that they help us think about the options facing adolescent parents, especially mothers. Using them, we will discuss responses that society can present to, advocate for, or discourage in young people coping with adolescent sexuality.

Diversity in the Data

Statistical trends this past decade in levels of adolescent sexual activity, contraceptive use, pregnancy, and childbirth illustrate both the inconsistency in progress toward pregnancy prevention and the diversity of patterning across social groups. Data from the third and fourth cycles of the National Surveys of Family Growth (NSFG) show that successively larger numbers of teenage women were exposed to the risks of early pregnancy during the 1980s. The number of adolescents aged fifteen to seventeen who ever had sexual intercourse rose from an estimated 33 percent in 1982 to 38 percent in 1988. Among adolescents aged eighteen to nineteen, the estimated rise was from 64 to 74 percent (Forrest and Singh 1990).

If other factors had remained unchanged, this rise in adolescent sexual activity would normally have translated into higher levels of teenage pregnancy. This did not happen because adolescent contraceptive practice improved, in the aggregate, during the 1980s. According to data from the NSFG, the proportions of sexually active teens who were currently practicing some form of contraception rose from an estimated 51 percent in 1982 to 60 percent in 1988 (Forrest and Singh 1990).[1] The cumulative effect, therefore, was one of little change in adolescent pregnancy rates, which hovered around an estimated 110 pregnancies per 1,000 women aged fifteen to nineteen years (Henshaw et al. 1991).

But the aggregate data blur the sometimes sharp distinctions between the experiences of different races and ethnic groups. The NSFG data indicate that the increase in female adolescent sexual activity was confined entirely to whites. The proportion of girls aged fifteen to nineteen who ever had sexual intercourse increased for non-Hispanic whites from 45 to 52 percent between 1982 and 1988, while it remained virtually unchanged for blacks at about 60 percent. Among Hispanic adolescents, sexual activity declined slightly to under 50 percent in 1988 (Forrest and Singh 1990).

While racial differences in levels of sexual activity narrowed during

TABLE 1.1.

Percent Change in Rates of Sexual Behaviors and Outcomes, 15–19-Year-Old Girls, 1982, 1987, 1988

	SEXUAL ACTIVITY 1982–88	CONTRACEPTION AT FIRST INTERCOURSE 1982–88	PREGNANCY 1982–87	ABORTION 1982–87	BIRTH 1982–87
Total	+13%	+36%	−1%	+1%	−4%
White	+16%	+26%	−5%	−5%	−7%
Nonwhite	—	—	+4%	+11%	−1%
Black	+3%	+50%	—	—	+3%

Sources: Rates of sexual activity and contraception at first intercourse are from Forrest and Singh (1990). They report rates for non-Hispanic whites and non-Hispanic blacks only. Rates for pregnancy and abortion are from Henshaw, Koonin, and Smith (1991). They do not separate out data on Hispanic whites or Hispanic blacks. Birthrates are from National Center for Health Statistics (1990). NCHS does not distinguish Hispanic from non-Hispanic whites or non-Hispanic blacks in its reporting. Empty cells result from sources' different reporting of data on nonwhites.

the 1980s, racial disparities in pregnancy rates for fifteen- to nineteen-year-olds widened. The pregnancy rate for whites decreased from 95 per 1,000 girls in 1982 to 90 per 1,000 in 1987 (Henshaw et al. 1991), despite an increase in sexual activity. The adolescent pregnancy rate for nonwhites rose from a low of 181 pregnancies per 1,000 girls in 1982 to 189 per 1,000 in 1987. Since their sexual activity level did not increase, the increase in the pregnancy rate leads to the inference that contraceptive practice lessened in effectiveness among nonwhite adolescents (Henshaw et al. 1991). This is surprising, given that the reported use of contraceptives at first intercourse went up from 36 to 54 percent for non-Hispanic blacks by 1988 (Forrest and Singh 1990). Whether the nonwhite teenagers practiced contraceptive less consistently or less effectively is unclear at present (see Gibbs this volume).

The divergences in pregnancy rates between races would not necessarily result in a greater discrepancy between birthrates if abortion rates changed sufficiently. Between 1982 and 1987, the abortion rate for whites declined 5 percent, from 38 to 36 abortions per 1,000 girls (see table 1.1). For nonwhites it increased 11 percent to 73 abortions per 1,000 girls (Henshaw et al. 1991).

These changes yielded no convergence in birthrates. Between 1982 and 1987, birthrates for whites decreased from 45 to 42 births per 1,000 girls aged 15–19. Those for nonwhites hardly decreased at all—from 92 to 91 births per 1,000 girls.[2] By 1988 both groups exhibited an upturn in teenage birthrates, and in 1989 the whites' reached the highest level since 1974 and the nonwhites' since 1976. Steady additions since 1983 to the birthrate for black fifteen- to nineteen-year-olds reached sufficient magnitude in 1988 to raise the birthrate for all nonwhite teenagers. The birthrate for nonwhite girls remains over twice as high as that for whites of the same age (National Center for Health Statistics 1991).

Taking a Biopsychosocial Perspective

Adolescent parenthood in startling proportions confronts the United States. The figures just presented, except the proportion of sexually active, are well above the rates for other industrialized countries (Jones et al. 1985). These data have been used to validate calls for intervention in order to counteract life courses fraught with difficulties such as low birth weight and morbidity-prone babies, low rates of high school completion for teenage mothers (and in turn for their children), and long-term welfare dependency for their families. Assessing where and how to intervene in the tangle of decision points requires a broad perspective. We propose a biopsychosocial perspective (see Hamburg 1986; Lancaster and Hamburg 1986).

A biopsychosocial viewpoint requires most simply that human phenomena be regarded as having biological, psychological, and social aspects. Motherhood is not merely a biological phenomenon—it is also psychological and social. The biological aspect of adolescent motherhood includes abortion decisions, prenatal care, and maternal and infant health. The psychological aspect brings into play emotional responses, ranging from pride and self-assertion to helplessness and depression, and cognitive capacities, such as knowledge of contraception and safe health practices. The psychological also includes subjective perceptions, such as teenagers' understanding of social norms or their ideas of how they look to their friends. The social side of adolescent parenthood involves, at least, family structure, community resources, norms for social behavior, and structural issues related to employment, housing, and government funding. As we discuss responses to adolescent parenthood, we shall draw attention to interactions among its biological, psychological, and social aspects.

Review of findings on the subgroup of adolescent mothers under fifteen years old has led us to conclude that, despite their small number, the interaction of their biological, psychological, and social contexts renders them sufficiently different from older school-age mothers that they merit separate discussion. While we have not attempted a thorough and systematic exposition of the problems of these very young teenage mothers, we conclude that the effort to draw together the biopsychosocial aspects of their experience suggests some potentially fruitful lines of investigation, as well as specific elements to include in interventions designed for this age group. We shall attempt to highlight research supplying information on biopsychosocial interactions for each subgroup of adolescent mothers discussed.

There are three age markers, biological, chronological, and social. Across most of the lifespan they are highly synchronized and their distinctiveness is not apparent. In adolescence, however, they tend to separate and troubling discrepancies can appear. Modern societies emphasize chronological age as the key marker. It is a basic requirement for legal milestones, such as purchasing of alcohol, marrying without parental consent, voting, and joining the military. Chronological age does not necessarily match biological age, however, which depends on timing of pubertal change. For example, a girl who reaches menarche at age eleven is simultaneously older biologically and younger chronologically than a fourteen-year-old who has not yet begun to menstruate. Finally, social age refers to the normative ages at which society expects people to have achieved major cultural transitions, such as graduating from school, entering the work force, getting married, having a child, or retiring. If a person violates the age norms associated with these transitions by being "off-time," that is, too early or too late, social and personal costs accrue (Neugarten 1979). Adolescent parenthood is a prime example.

Adolescent parenthood not only is asynchronous with the social age for other transitions to adulthood, but also involves a complex interplay of social age with chronological and biological age. A downward trend in biological age over the last century and a half (Eveleth 1986) and an upward trend in social age have resulted in a longer adolescence in modern society and multiple possibilities for asynchrony of biological and social capacities. Chronological age no longer serves as a marker of biological and social readiness for adult functions. "Teenage motherhood," therefore, designates too wide an age band. Eighteen- and nineteen-year-old mothers have reached legal adulthood and had the opportunity to graduate from high school. Their situations differ in these fundamental ways from those of minors who are school-age mothers.

This chapter will focus on the adaptations to pregnancy of school-age girls as well as the interventions that seem advisable for them.

Adoption and Abortion

Two ways to avoid the potential difficulties posed by off-time motherhood for high school or junior high students are adoption and abortion. By relinquishing the role of mother, girls who have abortions or put their babies up for adoption free themselves to concentrate on the social tasks that mainstream American society has set for them—schooling, experimentation with activities and personal strengths and weaknesses, forming relationships with same- and opposite-sex peers (Hamburg 1986; Zimring this volume). About 40 percent of pregnant white girls aged fifteen to nineteen chose abortion during the 1980s. The number of girls choosing adoption has not received the same attention, but in 1982 it was only 4.6 percent of pregnant fifteen- to nineteen-year-olds (Voydanoff and Donnelly 1990).

The biological and social aspects of these two strategies for dealing with adolescent pregnancy can, with some care and attention, resolve themselves without lasting damage to the girls involved. Still, health professionals and social service agencies must recognize that young women need psychological support no matter which of these two options they select. Greater attention to primary prevention of further untimely pregnancies is warranted.

But many pregnant teenagers cannot bring themselves to make either of these choices; and media and policy concern about adolescent pregnancy and childbearing have often focused on those who accept biological motherhood.

Early Marriage

Another way to cope with the prospect—or actuality—of off-time motherhood is early marriage. Marriage unites the social statuses of marriage and child rearing in the traditional manner, but it deviates from the expected age for adult behaviors in modern industrialized countries and can compound a teenage parent's off-time status. Early marriage and childbearing is counter to the trends of role transitions for mainstream women, who increasingly enter the work force relatively early, delay marriage, and begin childbearing significantly later than did women in the middle of this century.

In 1989 about one-third of white mothers aged fifteen through seventeen were married at the birth of their child, as were about 4 percent of black mothers the same age. The proportion of married mothers fifteen through seventeen for all races was about 22 percent (National Center for Health Statistics 1991). This shows a decrease over the ratios for 1985, when 29 percent of fifteen- to seventeen-year-old mothers were married at their child's birth (Children's Defense Fund 1988), and 1982, when 35 percent of fifteen- to seventeen-year-old mothers were married at their child's birth (National Center for Health Statistics 1984).

The expected benefits of marriage for an adolescent mother include financial support from her husband (see Testa chap. 6, this volume) and perhaps his relatives in addition to her own. More secure financial status helps ensure better maternal and infant health and the establishment of an independent household. Ideally, marriage also expands the number of relatives on whom the parents can call for child care, advice, and encouragement.

Marriage as a response to teenage parenthood has its pitfalls, however. One lies in the divorce rate, high enough for all couples but even higher for people who marry in their teen years (Chase-Lansdale and Vinovskis 1987; Norton and Moorman 1987; Furstenburg 1988; Vinovskis and Chase-Lansdale 1988). Another drawback, perhaps not readily apparent, to marriage for adolescent mothers is that the formation of an independent household can leave mother and child more vulnerable to homelessness if the marriage dissolves (Illinois Caucus on Teenage Pregnancy 1986). Parents who did not want to support their daughter and her baby may have encouraged marriage and later find themselves loath to accept the economic burden of daughter and baby in the aftermath of her marital crisis.

A recent study also shows that married mothers are less likely to finish high school than are unmarried mothers (Upchurch and McCarthy 1990). This tendency to forgo school completion not only endangers the mother if she divorces but also adds to the strain on the whole family when the marriage endures, because her potential contribution to their financial well-being will be limited by her lack of educational attainment (O'Connell and Rogers 1984).

For a majority of young women early marriage has proven to be a temporary and unsatisfactory solution to adolescent motherhood. The immediate benefit is far outweighed by the foreclosure of life options by lack of education and underemployability.

Alternative Life Course

Forming a single parent, mother-headed household is another strategy for coping with adolescent parenthood. Recent data offer hope that a subset of poor, unmarried teenage mothers may reach their mid-twenties—when chronological, biological, and social ages can return to synchrony—only marginally worse off than they would have been had they delayed childbearing, relinquished motherhood, or married. The descriptions of this alternative life course (Hamburg 1986) originated in ethnographic studies of poor, urban, African American neighborhoods in the early 1970s (Ladner 1971; Stack 1974). More recently, these constructs are being tested in quantitative studies. (See Geronimus 1987 and Luker 1991 for reviews.) Adolescent childbearing has gained the potential to function as an adaptive pattern of life in conditions of great poverty where networks of kin assist each other in bearing the stresses of disadvantaged lives (Anderson 1990) in which schooling is inferior and job opportunities are not available until adulthood.

Ladner (1971) argues that the girls she studied in a very poor neighborhood of St. Louis in the mid- to late-1960s could refer to at least two cultural patterns for their life course. One reflected the beliefs of what Ladner calls the dominant culture. From this set of beliefs the girls constructed idealized dreams of high-school completion, employment, marriage, family formation, and a life of at least middle-class amenities. The other relied on images drawn from African American traditions including women as the strong centers of family life, motherhood at any age as an entrance into womanhood, and reliance on a kin network as help in raising and supporting a child while the mother prepares for employability.

Taken in conjunction with other studies, Ladner's work points to a semi-institutional pattern for young women in impoverished, urban, black neighborhoods: they remain single, continue their education in high school, rely on relatives for childcare, housing, and other financial support, and perhaps have another child after high school but before their mid-twenties, when they enter the workforce which then begins to open up to them (Anderson 1990; Burton 1990; Sullivan 1986).

Ladner (1971) holds that structural factors tended to draw girls she studied into the sequence of lifecourse transitions that plays out as an alternative cultural model. For example, unemployment created a shortage of marriageable men who could find steady full-time work. Anderson (1990) twenty years later reaffirms this observation and adds that joblessness limited the modes of self-assertion and pride open to males, who enhanced their self-esteem by becoming fathers.

Stack (1974) cites several of the same factors as affecting life courses of women she studied at approximately the same time in a similar neighborhood of another midwestern city: the constant intrusion of unemployment on attempts to prosper, the disruptive effects of job loss on steady male-female relationships and associated housing arrangements, the valuing of children by the community, and the readiness of kin to assist in raising them. Like Ladner, she does not praise early childbearing as an ideal, but she believes that the pattern of life associated with it allowed people to adapt as well as possible to a grim and fairly intransigent reality.

The community that Ladner (1971) studied in fact lamented the destructive impact of adolescent childbearing on the girls' prospects for realizing the more ideal lifecourse pattern and possibly escaping from intergenerational poverty. It did not, however, proscribe nonmarital sexual experience. Nor did it offer access to or understanding of birth control. The girls' peers often disapproved of contraception, while their boyfriends pressured them for sex. When the girls became pregnant, they realized that they confronted a situation with which many of their relatives and neighbors had learned to cope.

The most important means of survival for these girls and their babies was their kin network's acceptance of the infant. The reality that they experienced in their social context was that the baby was born to the whole kin network (Stack 1974; Sullivan 1986), although from the viewpoint of the dominant culture it was seen as only a single-mother household. Both Stack and Ladner (1971) record many examples of persons who referred to someone other than their biological mother as their "mama" because that other person had raised them.

The birth of the teenager's baby activates the kin network, including the father's relatives if he acknowledges paternity. People who may otherwise be minimally involved with the adolescent mother rally to support her when she gives birth. Sullivan (1986), in a study of teenage fathers in a primarily black, low-income neighborhood in the 1980s, describes a process of negotiation between prospective adolescent mother and father and their parents regarding the rights and responsibilities of both sides of the family. He outlines a typical arrangement when all are agreed on the advisability of keeping the baby: the young unwed father would "seek employment and make financial contributions, . . . provide some child care, usually with the assistance of his own kin, . . . [and if] the father should continue with his schooling, he was still expected to seek part-time employment" (16–17).

The benefits of an early childbearing strategy have not been apparent to the outside observer. However, by the time the teenage mother reaches her mid-twenties they can be substantial. The adolescent herself may believe that she gains most promptly from immediate admission to adult status in her proximate social group. The first public benefit lies in higher rates of school graduation for girls who continue to live with their families and have child care and other supports (Testa chap. 6, this volume). Familial encouragement to obtain prenatal care connects the mother with the health care system, otherwise costly and often inaccessible for the poor (Geronimus 1987). Unemployment among black adolescents stood around 50 percent in the late 1980s; therefore, adolescent childbearing became a rational choice since job options were mostly unavailable. By the time full-time employment was available to a poor African American mother, she was in her mid-twenties and had completed her fertility. Children born in her teens could help manage household responsibilities. They would also attend school on a full-time basis and the need for child care would have greatly diminished when the mother joined the work force (Millman and Hendershot 1980; Furstenberg et al. 1987). As the work of Furstenberg and his colleagues has shown, a significant percentage of black teenage mothers from very disadvantaged circumstances have managed, by their late twenties or early thirties, to achieve an adequate or even good living for themselves (Furstenberg et al. this volume).

When economic conditions impose stringent enough constraints on social mobility, the potential gains of conforming to the mainstream life pattern tend to disappear. A poor black woman who waits to have children until her mid-twenties may not have enough money to pay for child care while she works, even if she has earned a college degree (Geronimus 1987). The losses to the pool of marriageable men in poor African American communities because of incarceration, unemployment, and death remain a feature of the lives of older as well as young females (Gibbs 1988b; this volume), and are considered to be a major contribution to the high rates of out-of-wedlock childbearing. Finally, contrary to beliefs about the intrinsic harm due to early childbearing, a recent longitudinal study of the health of women in Harlem (Brunswick and Aidala 1991) shows that physical and psychological health are not directly associated with age of mother at first birth.[3] In fact, among African Americans birth outcomes for both mother and child are superior for births prior to the early twenties.

A major drawback of the alternative life course is its effect on the child (or children). They are typically raised under conditions of poverty and deprivation in their formative early childhood and elementary school years. Although the majority make reasonable progress toward independent adulthood, there have been consistent findings of higher than average rates of behavioral problems and enduring deficits in school achievement among a substantial minority (Furstenberg et al. 1987, this volume). A sizable number of children of adolescent mothers struggle with the consequences of early childbearing.

Although the investigations that generated a comprehension of this potentially viable life course focused on urban poor black girls, it seems possible that disadvantaged girls in other ethnic subcultures may be negotiating similar life courses. Data show that poverty is the single best predictor of adolescent parenthood (Children's Defense Fund 1988). Petersen and Crockett (this volume) report studies of a subculture of poor white girls in rural areas that indicate patterns of adolescent sexuality and childbearing similar to those of the urban black adolescents. However, the patterns of kin support and long-term outcomes for the teenage mothers and their children in these white rural populations have not yet been studied.

Factors Affecting Motherhood at Less Than Fifteen Years Old

Although only 2 percent of births to teenagers and 0.3 percent of all births are to early adolescents (National Center for Health Statistics 1991), interventions to assist the very young girls cannot be targeted intelligently if we confound their cases with those of their older teenage counterparts. Adolescent mothers fourteen or younger cannot be expected to profit by putting child rearing in the context of marriage or of the alternative life course. While an average of 7 percent were married when they became mothers in the late 1980s, (National Center for Health Statistics, 1989, 1990, 1991), the quality of these marriages is in doubt. When childbearing begins very early there is a much longer time in their teen years during which these girls are at risk of having additional children. This heavy burden of parenthood militates against a successful negotiation of the alternative life course outlined above. In 1989, almost 400 of the births to girls less than fifteen years old were already second or later births (National Center for Health Statistics 1991).

Early adolescents experience a transition in social roles from grammar school child to junior high student that is typically associated with psychological stress. In the United States the entry into junior high school is the marker for entry into adolescent status. The early adolescents confront crucial emotionally charged decisions about the kind of person they want to be, how to make friends in junior high school, what to do about peer pressures to engage in risky behaviors such as smoking, drinking alcohol, or having sexual relations. Many of these are "hot" cognitions—thought processes invested with emotion and usually involving some anxiety, perception of threat, or conflict with cherished goals or values. For persons at all levels of intelligence and cognitive development, hot cognitions greatly impair information processing and decision making (Janis and Mann 1977). Not only are early adolescents likely to exhibit cognitive impairments in these circumstances, they also have not developed the formal operational thought that helps older teenagers and adults attain some measure of skill and objectivity in decision making (Neimark 1975; Berzonsky 1978). Moreover, young teenagers are prone to believe in a "personal fable" of invulnerability (Elkind 1981).

The outcome of these psychological immaturities may be reflected in their health care decisions. The data on initiation of prenatal care show that in recent years just over one-third of mothers under fifteen started prenatal care in the first trimester of pregnancy, and at least a fifth started it in the last trimester or failed to obtain prenatal care at all (National Center for Health Statistics 1989, 1990, 1991). While adolescence per se does not jeopardize maternal and infant health, both mother and infant are at higher risk without early attention from health professionals (Geronimus 1987). A study of vital statistics data in New York (1983–1985) showed that delayed prenatal care and infrequent visits approximately double the odds of a woman's delivering a low-birth-weight infant, regardless of maternal age, education, race, or the number of her previous births (New York State Department of Health 1989).

Although American society treats the teenage years as a time of growing autonomy, ten- to fourteen-year-olds are not prepared for the same independence as older youth. Many parents confuse the standards appropriate for junior high students with the proper limits for high school juniors and seniors and thereby fail to provide adequate guidance for young teenagers. Although early adolescents need to make trial-and-error experiments in their interactions with the larger world, adolescent sexuality is a dangerous field for such experimentation. On average 24 percent of all sexually active ten- to fourteen-year-olds are reported to become pregnant each year (Hofferth and Hayes 1987). In 1987, while only 10,311 girls under fourteen years old had babies, another 16,090 had abortions (Henshaw et al. 1991).

The immaturity of the girls' cognitive capabilities, their emotional vulnerability in puberty and at the beginning of junior high school, and the ages of their sexual partners combine to raise the question of how much sexual activity at this age is truly consensual. The onset of puberty in themselves and their classmates can keep sex highly charged if only vaguely comprehended for most young teenage girls, and older boys may make advances to younger girls whom they find attractive. Moore and her colleagues report that 5.8 percent of white women and 2.0 percent of black women between the ages of eighteen and twenty-two reported having had nonvoluntary sexual intercourse when they were less than fourteen years old. Another 6.3 percent and 3.2 percent, respectively, reported nonvoluntary sexual intercourse by the time they reached fifteen (Moore et al. 1989).

In another study, the average age of first occurrence of coercive sexual experience reported by women who became mothers in adolescence was 11.5 years (Gershenson et al. 1989). A full 24 percent of the mothers surveyed reported that they had been forced to have sexual intercourse with the first perpetrator of abuse and 33 percent indicated ever having been forced to have intercourse. Another 28 percent reported some other unwanted sexual experience. Petersen and Crockett (this volume; see also Gershenson et al. 1989) mention mechanisms by which coercive sexual experience prior to puberty could affect the abused child's sexual activity in her early teen years.

Psychosocial theory suggests that a subset of mothers of this age may represent a more problem-prone group. Sexual and pregnancy behaviors of many adolescents have been shown to be correlated with other adolescent problem behaviors such as alcohol consumption, drug use, and poor school achievement. Jessor and Jessor (1975) have suggested that engaging in problem behavior serves important functions for adolescents that may include: (1) an effort to achieve otherwise unavailable goals; (2) a learned way of coping with personal frustrations and anticipated failure; (3) an expression of opposition to or rejection of conventional society; (4) a negotiation for accelerated transition to adulthood; or (5) a badge of membership in peer subculture. Their theory of "problem-proneness" (1977) holds that personality and social environment interact to set regulatory norms that define age-appropriate behaviors for individuals. The likelihood of an adolescent's adhering to these age norms depends on the balance among instigations by peers and role models, the maturity of personal controls, and psychosocial orientations with respect to social supports and expectations of others, particularly parents. Problem proneness may also be associated with psychiatric disorder such as depression or conduct disorder. There has been little systematic investigation in these areas.

Interventions

The considerations presented thus far demonstrate that no single etiology underlies the recently rising incidence of adolescent parenthood.

Yet the single factor of poverty stands behind two threats to the well-being of young girls who are most likely to conceive or bear children: lack of opportunity to obtain a good education and pessimistic expectations about present or future employment that pays a living wage (compare Ladner 1971; see Children's Defense Fund 1987a, 1988; Anderson 1990). These are issues that mediate the relationship of poverty to adolescent parenthood (Belle 1982). Programs that reach out to young fathers, as well as mothers, to help them learn responsible parenthood and assist them with job training and job search are essential for improving physical, psychological, and social outcomes for early parents and their children.

Our concern with opportunity implicates government because of the magnitude of the problem and its embeddedness in the structure of our economy. State and federal programs intended to assist the least advantaged populations must take cognizance of the role of opportunity in helping people short-circuit the problems associated, as either cause or effect, with adolescent parenthood (Children's Defense Fund 1988). The Family Support Act of 1988 takes into account many school-age parents' need for services that will enable them to complete high school and learn job skills. This often entails day care for the child or children as part of the program of training and employment. Unfortunately, lack of funding for social programs has limited numbers of eligible persons who actually are provided services.

The first goal of interventions targeted to the specific problem of adolescent pregnancy should be to the postponement of sexual intercourse for both males and females to a later age, and the responsible use of contraceptives starting with the initial sexual encounter. The rise in adolescent sexual activity may have to do partly with the lack of clear guidelines in our society about the appropriate age for becoming sexually active or about the use of contraceptives.

A kindergarten-through-twelfth-grade school curriculum of health and sex education appears to be the most promising primary prevention approach. An awareness of the development of children's cognitive and social capacities should underlie it. More complex and detailed information should enter the lessons year by year in accordance with the developmental stage of the individual. Repetition of the most crucial facts and ideas ought to be sequenced to yield a "booster" effect as the child develops. The increased use of condoms by adolescents, largely in response to the concern about AIDS, gives encouragement to the assumption that with appropriate information and guidance adolescents can and will make safe choices.

Various programs of training in life skills offer a method of teaching responsible decision making and enhancing social competence to carry out personal intentions (Hamburg 1990). Young people with training in life skills learn to formulate and implement their own intentions in conjunction with the counsel of trusted adults, preferably including parents. Life skills could help disaffected youngsters come to terms with conflicting social expectations, preserve their racial or ethnic identity, and at the same time acquire the motivation and skills to succeed in mainstream society. Finally, such skills seem crucial for young adolescent girls who may have tried to "just say no" to no avail. They need assertiveness training and role plays to help them state and maintain refusal in sexual encounters.

The second goal of intervention should be to provide those adolescents who are already sexually active with birth control information and access to contraceptive services. Much of this has been done in Planned Parenthood clinics with an almost exclusively female clientele. School-based clinics have also proved themselves as sources of health care where birth control and pregnancy referral information is available. Although these clinics have generated some controversy, communities with high levels of teenage pregnancy have in general strongly supported them. In addition, recent outreach efforts to include males (Dryfoos 1988) should increase in number and prominence.

The third goal of intervention should be to provide services and support to adolescents who are pregnant and expecting to give birth. For them, the most effective programs are those that encourage and provide early, sustained, and comprehensive prenatal care. The value of high-quality prenatal care is firmly established. There is still a challenge to reach the youngest mothers, who have proven to be most in need but most inaccessible.

A fourth goal should be psychological assessment with specific treatment for conduct disorder, depression, or other psychiatric disorders (Hamburg 1986; Coletta 1983).

This description of interventions does not exhaust the relevant possibilities.

Systematic evaluation of programs should be emphasized, and attention should be paid to the ingredients that facilitate constructive adaptations of young parents and enable them to achieve ordinary expectable or "good enough" results for themselves and their infants. We need to learn what works for women and which elements of the newer, more intensive and comprehensive programs contribute most to success. Comprehensive programs generally have higher costs than earlier, more focused efforts, but the expense follows predictably from the larger effort to address simultaneously the related problems of providing not only health care but also resources to meet the educational, vocational, and psychological needs of young people preparing successfully to fulfill adult roles as parents and workers.

Our counterpart industrial nations have shown us that even in postindustrial societies where the traditional roles of women have changed and sexual freedom has increased, adolescent pregnancy and childbearing have been constrained (see Hoem this volume; Jones et al. 1985, 1986). We can learn from them. We must also learn from our own examined experience as we try to address a complex issue with preventive interventions that meet adolescent needs which, while many and diverse, are neither infinite nor intractable.

NOTES

1. These figures on contraceptive use among sexually active teens were calculated by a method suggested by William Mosher, statistician with the Family Growth Survey Branch of the National Center for Health Statistics (personal communication). They are based on NSFG data reported in tables 1 and 3 in Forrest and Singh (1990) and in table 4 in Mosher (1990). According to these data, 4,883,000, or 53.2 percent, of the 9,179,000 women aged fifteen to nineteen in 1988 in the United States ever had sexual intercourse. An estimated 2,950,000 women aged fifteen to nineteen were currently practicing some form of contraception in 1988. Dividing these two figures (2,950,000/4,883,000) yields an estimate of 60 percent of sexually active teens currently practicing some form of contraception in 1988. The 1982 estimate of 51.3 percent was calculated in the same way using the corresponding figures from the 1982 NSFG.

2. Data for years prior to 1989 used the race of the child to stand for the race of the mother when reporting births. When reporting rates of births per 1,000 teenage girls of a given age group, however, the denominator was based on the number of girls of the race and age in question. The resulting discrepancy of determination of race in numerator (race of child) and denominator (race of

mother) will disappear eventually because the National Center for Health Statistics has begun to use the race of the mother in the numerator to calculate birth rates (National Center for Health Statistics 1991).

For the 1989 data, figures based on both race of mother and race of child were reported. The birthrates based on race of mother were about 3 percent higher than the birthrates based on race of child for whites aged fifteen to nineteen. For nonwhites aged fifteen to nineteen, birthrates based on race of mother were about 5 percent lower than those based on race of child. For blacks the race of mother yielded a birthrate about 4 percent lower in the same age range. For the purpose of historical comparisons in this paper we continue to use the race of child to stand for the race of mother.

3.   The major factor distinguishing outcomes was not age at childbearing but heroin use, which was correlated with early parenthood. Provided no addiction to heroin entrapped them, the women who waited to bear children were as well—or as badly—off, except in educational attainment, as those who first gave birth as teenagers.

ANNE C. PETERSEN and LISA J. CROCKETT

2   Adolescent Sexuality, Pregnancy, and Child Rearing: Developmental Perspectives

Over the past three decades there have been striking changes in patterns of teenage sexual activity, pregnancy, and childbearing. In part these trends are attributable to larger societal changes related to sex, marriage, and childbearing, but they may also reflect changes specific to adolescence and adolescent development. We review the demographic trends briefly and then turn to several developmental factors that may affect adolescent sexuality, pregnancy, and child-rearing competence.

Demographic Trends

As noted in other chapters, beginning in the 1960s the incidence of sexual activity among teenagers increased dramatically. The increase in adolescent sexual activity, together with a trend toward later marriage, contributed to a rise in premarital pregnancy during the 1970s (Furstenberg and Brooks-Gunn 1986). Despite this rise, teen birthrates actually decreased over the same period, due to the increased use of abortion (Hayes 1987). Nonetheless, teenage pregnancy gained national visibility because the births that resulted frequently occurred out of wedlock. The increase in the proportion of nonmarital births among teenagers, along with adolescents' increased use of abortion, focused public concern on adolescent pregnancy and childbearing.

The 1960s–1990s in the United States has been a period characterized by delayed transitions to traditional adult work and family roles, as indicated by later age at marriage and postponement of full-time employment. The delayed transition to adulthood has meant an extension of the adolescent period. At the same time, the onset of puberty, which is usually taken as the beginning of adolescence, has been occurring at younger and younger ages over the past century (Tanner 1972). Thus, there is evidence that adolescence represents an expanded period of life in contemporary technological society. Indeed, growing numbers of adolescents are continuing secondary and postsecondary schooling and, therefore, dependent adolescent roles. It is noteworthy that most developmentalists now define adolescence as the second decade of life—a ten-year period.

Traditionally, the transition to adulthood has involved a sequence of events consisting of completion of schooling, perhaps some work experience, marriage, and then childbearing (Hogan 1982*a*). In contemporary society teenage childbearing disrupts this sequence, because adolescent mothers typically enter their new family roles before entering work roles and often before completion of schooling. The implications for the institutions of marriage and family are profound. The fact that adolescent childbearing is off-time and out of sequence may help account for the negative consequences early childbearing often has for the development and well-being of mother and child (Hayes 1987). Ultimately, however, the increased prevalence of this nontraditional sequence may alter our views of the normative developmental sequence.

Developmental Hypotheses

Currently, with relatively effective contraception and safe abortion techniques, sexual intercourse is no longer so closely linked to childbearing. Thus, intercourse, pregnancy, and childbearing are now more distinctly separable events. Girls who are sexually active earlier may or may not become pregnant; those who become pregnant may or may not go on to bear a child; and bearing a child does not have any necessary relation to competence in rearing a child. Accordingly, for each step in the sequence from adolescent intercourse to effective child rearing, there are likely to be different developmental predictors. In the sections that follow, we identify four hypotheses for developmental processes related to the outcomes of sexual activity, pregnancy, and child-rearing competence. These hypotheses include (1) biological influences; (2) results of prepubertal sexual abuse; (3) engaging in deviant or problem behavior; and (4) effects of norms or expectations for the life course.

Biological Effects of Puberty

Puberty has been proposed as a major influence on adolescent sexual behavior, creating the risk of premarital pregnancy and childbearing. Pubertal development may affect adolescent sexuality in two ways: directly, through hormonal effects on the brain; and indirectly, through somatic changes that lead to the development of a mature physical appearance, which in turn triggers expectations for more mature behavior. Some evidence exists for each of these processes. Hormonal stimulation of adolescent sexual behavior is supported by the finding that androgen levels are related to sexual motivation and noncoital sexual experience in adolescents of both sexes, and also to coital experience in boys (Udry et al. 1985, 1986). Indirect pubertal effects are suggested by findings that more physically mature girls are perceived as more attractive by boys (see, e.g., Simmons and Blyth 1987) and may thus have more opportunities for sexual involvement (Udry et al. 1986).

Pubertal status effects, which may reflect both hormonal influences and attractiveness, have also been documented. Morris, Mallin, and Udry (1982) found associations between specific pubertal characteristics and recent intercourse, although the relationships varied by sex and race. They were strongest for white males and black females and weakest for black males. The lack of relationship for black males is underscored by the finding that many of these boys report prepubertal coital experience (Udry 1982). In our own research we find strong relationships between pubertal status and cross-sex activities such as dating and "making out," especially among girls (Crockett and Petersen 1987). Models that include both peer influences and biological factors, however, appear to provide the most powerful prediction of adolescent sexual behavior (Billy and Udry 1985).

An important trend alluded to earlier is the secular trend in timing of puberty. As Tanner and others have demonstrated, menarche has occurred about two to three months earlier each decade over the past century (see, e.g., Eveleth 1986). Some investigators have also examined age at peak height velocity (i.e., peak growth rate during the adolescent growth spurt), an indicator equally relevant for boys and girls (see, e.g., Marshall and Tanner 1969, 1970). A similar decline in age has been found with this indicator, suggesting that puberty in general, and not just the onset of reproductive potential in girls, is occurring earlier. Most scholars attribute this to improved nutrition and health, reflecting an improved standard of living. In recent years the trend seems to have leveled off.

Some scholars have hypothesized that the secular trend in age at puberty underlies the recent trends in adolescent sex and pregnancy. As we have noted previously, however, these two sets of trends do not match (Petersen and Boxer 1982). The secular trend in age at menarche has been advancing at a rate of about two to three months per decade over the past century, whereas the increase in sexual activity was seen in the 1970s and 1980s and primarily in white females.

A distinct but related question is whether pubertal maturation influences child-rearing competence. In a previous paper (Petersen and Crockett 1986), we examined three hypotheses related to pubertal effects on adolescent child-rearing competence. We pursued these hypotheses because one could argue that the advent of pubertal change brings with it effects on other aspects of functioning. These three hypotheses were described as generalized maturation, pubertal disruption, and perimenarcheal enhancement. In a generalized maturation model, cognitive and psychosocial maturity are assumed to be a function of physiological or reproductive maturity. For example, it is possible that pubertal development is related to brain maturation, and that pubertal brain maturation permits the emergence of abstract reasoning. Similarly, the mature biological status of postmenarcheal girls, because it marks the completion of the biological transition, could lead to a more integrated self-image as well as greater social status. If the generalized maturation model were correct, we would see positive linear relationships between reproductive maturity and cognitive and psychosocial maturity. Girls reaching puberty early would be no more at risk than later maturers in terms of their degree of cognitive and psychosocial maturity, because cognitive and psychosocial competence would develop at the same time as reproductive competence.

In the pubertal disruption model, it is assumed that there is a period of disruption in the lives of young girls as they become biologically mature. We know that the development of a mature menstrual cycle is a lengthy process in which menarche is but a single event (Petersen 1979, 1983; Petersen and Taylor 1980). The endocrine changes associated with this process could directly disrupt cognition and psychological functioning and consequently affect cognitive performance and social relationships.

If this pubertal disruption model were correct, we would see concave curvilinear relationships between menarcheal age and cognitive or psychosocial measurements such that performance would be lowest for girls currently in the midst of pubertal change. Therefore, girls who have recently begun menstruation would be at particular risk as child-rearers.

Models showing the opposite predictions from those described above could be proposed on logical and empirical grounds. We could argue that puberty brings with it a general deterioration, rather than a general improvement in competence. For example, some of the data on the development of sex differences (see, e.g., Maccoby and Jacklin 1974; Petersen 1980) would suggest that, beginning in early adolescence, girls start to decrease their rate of growth in achievement, decline in self-esteem, and are at increased risk for depression. Such phenomena could be part of an underlying process of maturationally based decline. This hypothesis is a variant of the generalized maturation model; the only difference is the negative slope of the line.

Similarly, the converse of the pubertal disruption model is a pubertal enhancement model. There is little theoretical or empirical support for such a model, although one could argue that increased pubertal hormones temporarily enhance some behavioral processes. Belief in hypersexuality during early adolescence would be consistent with this model. Evidence for this model would fit a convex curve peaking at mid-puberty.

On the basis of research testing these hypotheses (Petersen and Crockett 1986), we concluded that advances in cognitive capacity and psychosocial functioning occur over the course of adolescence. Few links, however, were found between reproductive maturation and these advances. Instead, very strong relationships were found with chronological age. Increasing menarcheal age was related to only a few cognitive and achievement measures. No evidence was found in our data for a maturationally based decline in functioning. Support for the hypotheses of pubertal disruption or enhancement (i.e., curvilinear patterns) was found with a few variables, but at a frequency similar to that expected by chance. We concluded that age-related advances and experience, rather than biological development, appear to affect the child-rearing capacities of adolescent girls. By implication, the same could be said of young girls' capacities to make wise decisions about sex, pregnancy, and childbearing. A sixth-grade girl is much less mature, both cognitively and psychosocially, than a twelfth-grade girl. When the increase in experience gained over these years is also considered, the case is even stronger for greater competence in older adolescents. Young adolescent girls, particularly those under fifteen years, appear more likely to be poor mothers, given a significantly less mature developmental status. Although cognitive and psychosocial competence cannot guarantee adequate child-rearing competence, they at least make it more likely.

In summary, although current hypotheses would predict positive effects of pubertal hormones and status on adolescent fertility behavior, the research finds effects only for sexuality. Except for the obvious requirement of reproductive maturity for pregnancy, effects of pubertal hormones and status on the likelihood of becoming pregnant and on child-rearing competence are unlikely, according to current research.

Sexual Abuse

Trickett and Putnam (1987) have recently hypothesized that prepubertal sexual abuse has significant effects on the subsequent pubertal development and sexual behavior of girls. They propose three distinct hypotheses: (1) amplification of normal pubertal effects; (2) elevated adrenal or gonadotrophic hormones; and (3) preferential development and preservation of dissociative capacity. They posit that puberty is likely to stimulate a recapitulation of prior abuse trauma, therefore making the pubertal experience more difficult. In addition, they hypothesize that pubertal effects will be amplified because most of these youngsters lack full family support for typical developmental challenges, particularly the ones bringing increased autonomy. Finally, they propose that girls sexually abused before puberty are more likely to be early maturers, a factor found in other research to be related to greater difficulty in traversing the pubertal period (e.g., Tobin-Richards et al. 1983; Magnusson et al. 1985; Simmons and Blyth 1987). In contrast to most speculation that early maturers provoke sexual abuses, these researchers posit the reverse causal direction: that early pubertal maturation is related to elevated hormone levels stimulated by the earlier sexual involvement. The elevated hormone levels, in turn, could influence inappropriate sexual behavior and aggression. Trickett and Putnam also hypothesize that sexually abused girls will, as a result of the abuse, manifest a learning disability or at least poor concentration capacity as well as poor self-esteem. These hypotheses are currently being examined in an ongoing, well-designed study (Trickett and Putnam 1987); preliminary results show clear effects in the hypothesized direction (Putnam 1990; Trickett et al. 1990).

Burton and her students (see, e.g., Butler 1988) have also studied sexual abuse in relation to some of the issues of interest here. In a study in eastern Pennsylvania, Butler (1988) found that 54 percent of white adolescent mothers had been sexually abused. These investigators speculate that sexual abuse played a causal role in the adolescent pregnancies, with some girls intentionally becoming pregnant to escape their current situations and another group unintentionally becoming pregnant as a result of promiscuity and engagement in other problem behaviors. The two groups were both likely to suffer from feelings of low self-worth and may be more similar than different psychologically. Low self-esteem may also be related to the decision to keep the baby, since some girls acknowledge wanting a child who will love them.

Although there has been little research on the effects of sexual abuse on adolescent child-rearing, research with adults who were abused as children suggests that such experience impairs the development of good child-rearing capacity. Egeland et al. (1988), for example, found that mothers who had been physically abused as children were more likely to abuse their own children. In addition, girls may enter other abusive relationships, exposing themselves and their babies to stressful and even dangerous conditions.

In summary, it has been hypothesized that prepubertal sexual abuse is linked to earlier sexual experience, earlier pregnancy, earlier childbearing, and poorer child-rearing skills. Although research examining these hypotheses is very limited, there is modest support for them.

Deviance or Problem Behavior

Precocious or excessive involvement in adult behaviors (e.g., drinking, drug use) during adolescence, often called problem behavior, has been hypothesized as leading to earlier sexual behavior and earlier pregnancy. Indeed, some scholars argue that adolescent sexual activity is part of a problem behavior syndrome (Jessor and Jessor 1977). Several other behaviors have increased over the past two decades, parallel to the rise in sexual activity. Examples include juvenile delinquency, suicide, and running away, with only drug use showing a somewhat different pattern of increase and then recent decrease (Johnston et al. 1987). Elliott (in press) provides evidence that sexual behavior, substance use, and delinquency tend to co-occur, thus supporting the hypothesis of at least a related pattern of behavior, if not a syndrome. This hypothesis, as well as the (next) one focused on normative expectations for early transitions to adult roles, form the major hypotheses of a current study on rural adolescents.

This study (Vicary 1985) hypothesizes that both the problem behavior patterns and the normative expectations pattern will predict early sexual activity and pregnancy. The study involves a longitudinal design in which three cohorts of youngsters initially seen in grades seven through nine are followed for five years. Assessments include an annual fall survey of all students in these cohorts in an entire school district, spring interviews with girls at high and low risk for early pregnancy based on deviance and normative risk factors, and pregnancy and postpartum interviews with girls who become pregnant. The community in which these hypotheses are pursued is rural, low to middle income, and white. Based on 1980 census data, only 7 percent of the adults had completed college, and another 44 percent had completed high school. The median household income was $14,500 in 1980; the modal occupations were those of laborers and technicians or clerical workers.

In these data, both mild delinquency and substance use significantly differentiate pre- and post-coital groups of girls. We have examined the mean reported frequency of mild delinquency, being drunk, and being high on drugs. In each case, the means are higher for nonvirgins than for virgins. These factors, taken together, significantly predict the onset of sexual behavior in a regression analysis (unpublished data).

A relationship between problem behavior and early sexual activity has also been documented in other research. Alcohol use, cigarette smoking, and illicit drug use, as well as delinquent behavior, have been found to correlate with precocious sexual activity (e.g., Jessor and Jessor 1977; Ensminger 1987). In addition, recent factor analytic studies suggest that behaviors such as frequent excessive drinking, marijuana use, sexual intercourse, and general deviance (antisocial behaviors) load on a common factor for adolescents and young adults (Donovan and Jessor 1985).

At least two processes may help account for the relationship between early sexual activity and other problem behaviors. First, as suggested by the Jessors (Jessor and Jessor 1977), involvement in problem behaviors may indicate psychological readiness to engage in adult behaviors, or "transition-proneness." Second, engagement in one type of problem behavior may bring adolescents into contact with peer groups or peer activities in which other problem behaviors are modeled and encouraged (Donovan and Jessor 1985). In either case, we would expect participation in substance use or deviance to predict the onset of sexual activity in the near future. This is what we find in our rural adolescent data.

A recent review (Elliott, in press) notes that there is some evidence of a relationship between early pregnancy and both drug use and delinquency. Elliott concludes that premarital pregnancy appears to be part of the "deviant life-style," a life-style characterized by multiple problem behaviors. There appears to be no clear evidence linking problem behaviors to childbearing or child-rearing competence, however.

Normative Expectations

Our final developmental hypothesis stems from life-span theory (e.g., Baltes et al. 1980; Elder 1985). Within this framework, transitions to subsequent life stages are thought to be largely influenced by societal or subcultural expectations (i.e., normative expectations) for appropriate timing. For example, if an adolescent's parents expect the adolescent to complete college before making other transitions (e.g., to marriage or full-time employment), this adolescent is more likely to complete his or her education in the early twenties, begin full-time work, and then marry and have children. This sequence of expectations has been considered the normative model for college-bound youth (Hogan 1982a), although other sequences have been documented (Rindfuss et al. 1987). The pattern among adolescents completing their schooling earlier typically follows the same sequence but involves making the transitions at earlier ages. Girls expecting to complete only high school studies typically have less invested in a career role and expect to get married and bear children shortly after graduation. The recent trend toward earlier and premarital pregnancy reverses these sequences (Hogan 1982a).

In the rural adolescent study described, we found associations between sexual behaviors and factors reflecting expectations for early transitions to adult roles. Girls who become sexually active in junior high anticipated making several adult transitions (finishing their full-time education, starting their first full-time job, marrying, and becoming a mother) at earlier ages than did girls who were not yet sexually active (unpublished data). In addition, there was evidence of familial transmission of these expectations; for example, mother's age at the birth of her first child was rather strongly related to her adolescent daughter's level of sexual experience. Other normative factors—such as the experience of having a sister who was pregnant as an adolescent or anticipating only a high school education—were less dramatically related to level of sexual experience in these girls. Notably, the differences between virgins and nonvirgins decreased at later times of measurement when being sexually active was more common.

A relationship between low educational aspirations and early onset of sexual activity has been documented in other research (Chilman 1986; Miller and Sneesby 1988). The other normative risk factors discussed here have been examined only infrequently in the empirical literature on adolescent sex, pregnancy, and childbearing (see Hayes 1987, or Petersen et al. 1988, for a review.) Hogan and Kitagawa (1985) reported a relationship between having a sister who was pregnant as a teen and a girl's likelihood of being sexually active and getting pregnant. In addition, a relationship has been found between mothers' reported level of sexual experience as teenagers and the sexual experience of their adolescent sons and daughters (Newcomer and Udry 1984; Udry and Billy 1987). It has been suggested (Fox 1981) that the key to this connection is a permissive attitude about sex that is passed on from mother to child. Similarly, a greater familial tolerance about early sex and childbearing could explain the association found in our rural study between mother's age at first birth and daughter's sexual activity. An alternative explanation may involve the correlation between timing of puberty in mothers and their children: since early maturers tend to begin sexual activity at a younger age, correlated timing of puberty could help explain the relationship between mother's and daughter's sexual (and pregnancy) experience (e.g., Newcomer and Udry 1984). Normative factors may also help explain the well-documented relationship between low SES and early sexual activity (e.g., Bolton 1980; Hogan and Kitagawa 1985; Robbins et al. 1985).

Examination of the pregnancy data from our rural sample suggests that the normative factors are important risk indicators for early pregnancy and childbearing. Currently, fifty-one pregnant girls have been identified. Over three-quarters (76%) of these girls have at least one of the normative risk factors under study (i.e., a mother who was a teenage parent, a sister who became pregnant as a teen, or low educational goals). For example, the pregnant girls' mothers had their first child at just under twenty years of age, on average, compared to age twenty-one for mothers of nonpregnant girls. In addition, 35 percent of the pregnant girls with sisters had sisters who were pregnant as teens compared to 17 percent among other girls. Finally, girls who became pregnant had lower educational plans than those who did not become pregnant; they were less likely to plan to attend college even before becoming pregnant. When we compared pregnant girls who had live births (early mothers) with those who chose to terminate the pregnancy, childbearers were more likely to have had mothers who became parents before age twenty and were more likely to have anticipated only a high school education prior to pregnancy. There were no differences in the proportions with sisters who were pregnant as teens. Although the samples were small (data were based on twenty-three live births and seven abortions), the results implicate at least two normative factors in a pregnant adolescent's decision to bear a child. We have no data yet on child-rearing efficacy but note that familial norms favorable to early childbearing could lead to more support.

In summary, we could hypothesize that normative expectations for earlier transitions to adult roles would lead to earlier sexual behavior, earlier pregnancy, earlier childbearing, and, possibly, more effective child-rearing, assuming that families expecting these early transitions are also willing to provide the necessary support. Thus far, the existing research suggests that these normative expectations may lead to earlier sexual experience and are likely to lead to earlier pregnancy and child-bearing. We have not yet examined effects on child-rearing competence.

Summary

We conclude that there may be different developmental pathways to early sexual behavior, pregnancy, childbearing, and child-rearing effectiveness among adolescents. Early sexual behavior appears to be related to earlier pubertal maturation, prior sexual abuse, problem behaviors such as drug or alcohol use and delinquency, and expectations for an earlier transition to adulthood. There is a hypothesis that earlier pregnancy and childbearing are related to these same factors, although the evidence is less available and clear. Child-rearing competence, in contrast, may reasonably be hypothesized to relate *negatively* to most of the factors that lead to early sex and pregnancy. Where evidence is available—and it is very sparse indeed—child-rearing competence appears to be unrelated or negatively related to factors leading to early sex or pregnancy. Adolescents who are expected by their families to bear children as teenagers may differ from this pattern, although more evidence is needed to confirm this hypothesis.

The relative lack of information on the child-rearing competence of adolescent mothers is surely related to the paucity of research generally on effective parenting. Literature on this topic is beginning to accumulate (e.g., Cohen et al. 1984; Lancaster et al. 1987), but strong feelings about the need for privacy within the home have made this a very difficult topic to study in many communities, even relative to other sensitive topics such as sexual behavior.

For many adolescent mothers, however, their challenge is made more complex because they are attempting to master two developmental tasks at once: adolescence and motherhood (Sadler and Catrone 1983). Especially because the demands of being an adolescent and those of being a mother are often divergent, the youngster who tries to be both at once may compromise one or the other, or fail at both. Because motherhood is irreversible, short of drastic measures, it may be easier to give up adolescence. Whether this can be done successfully—whether there are developmental losses involved in prematurely leaving adolescence—has not been examined empirically, to our knowledge, but we speculate that important learning and experience could be foreclosed by premature motherhood. The context in which earlier motherhood is expected and supported may, of course, minimize any developmental losses.

Some environments in which adolescent motherhood is fully expected, and even supported, may nevertheless be difficult environments for development. Many of our rural Appalachian families, for example, have histories of unemployment, alcohol problems, and family violence. Early pregnancy may be more likely in these families, but their broader problems compromise their effectiveness as development-enhancing environments for adolescents and their offspring. Growing up is difficult for many adolescents these days, but it is surely more difficult for some than others. Our research suggests that poor rural adolescents have significantly lower self-esteem and more depression than youngsters growing up in more privileged environments (Sarigiani et al. 1990).

Those subgroups of youngsters at higher risk for poor outcomes deserve special scrutiny in our research and programs. Rural youths, for example, have been neglected thus far in programs and research. Yet the evidence suggests that they are similar to poor urban youth in many respects. We need careful prediction models such as those being developed by Testa (chap. 6, this volume). We also need to pay attention to trends in these subgroups. Policy changes, such as in foster care and placement of youngsters who have been physically or sexually abused, are important to follow for effects on developmental outcomes.

Young people represent our future. It is in our best interest to ensure that our policies and practices enhance their development to the greatest extent possible. At the very least, we should attempt to minimize damage.

ANDREW M. BOXER

3 Adolescent Pregnancy and Parenthood in the Transition to Adulthood

Intervening effectively in adolescent pregnancy depends on an under-standing of socio-historical, cultural, and developmental factors affecting adolescents and their behavior. The life-course perspective (Elder 1975) relating developmental changes to social context provides a useful frame-work for studying adolescent sexuality and pregnancy. Additional impor-tant factors that influence adolescent development include historical time and important social structures, particularly families and schools. My comments address two critical issues: (1) teen sexuality and (2) research questions on adolescent parenting from a life-course perspective.

Adolescent Sexuality

Adolescent pregnancy is profitably viewed through attention to the sub-jective dimension of teen sexuality, sexual desire. Our understanding of, and ability to design interventions to prevent, adolescent pregnancy will continue to be impeded so long as we neglect this critical aspect of adoles-cent experience. In order to further our understanding of adolescent sex-uality, we must look beyond the simple quantification of its occurrence.[1]

Public schools have become a target for efforts to control and contain adolescent sexuality, which is typically viewed as a Freudian cauldron of out-of-control impulses. An implicit assumption of many school-based policies regarding sex education is that a causal relationship exists between discussions of sexuality, sexual desires or behaviors, and an increase in sexual activity. Empirical evidence does not support this assumption (see, e.g., Furstenberg et al. 1986).

Fine (1988) has argued that the way sexuality is defined in the school arena allows girls one critical decision, to say yes or no; the choice is defined as either engaging in sexual intercourse with a male or not. There is a "code of silence" (Gagnon 1989) about various forms of adolescent sexual behavior, including homosexuality and masturbation. Typically, sex is taught as the biology of reproduction. Youth may learn about the act of insemination or nocturnal emissions, but the sexual desires of females are far less often the topic of discussion (Fine 1988). Sex education in the public schools has typically represented adolescent females as lacking sexual desire. Males have typically been represented as singularly focused on obtaining sexual pleasure. Thus, discourse disproportionately focuses on female victimization. Fine has argued that this approach transforms anxieties about female sexuality into protective talk while derogating female desire. The outcome of this missing "discourse of desire" is that young teenage women are unable to negotiate their own sexual behavior and end up in positions of passivity and victimization (Fine 1988).

School-based definitions of the meaning of sexual coercion and consent for sexual behavior are typically organized around chronological age and marital status. Thus, women who represent female sexual subjectivities outside marriage, particularly single mothers, are excluded from the representations of female sexuality commonly portrayed in educational institutions. The general attitude conveyed is that women who are both reproductively "out of control" (e.g., have an unplanned pregnancy) and "in control" (practice successful contraception outside marriage) should all be viewed as out of control (Vance 1984; Gagnon 1989). It has been argued that the language of female victimization and the underlying concern for saying "no" to stop sexual behavior denies young women the right to control their own sexuality by depriving them of access to a legitimate sexual subjectivity.

Pregnancy prevention and sex education must acknowledge and discuss the fact that sex is pleasurable and exciting, because teenagers experience sex in this manner (Levinson 1984, 1986). Failure to orient instruction this way miseducates adolescents in general, and young teen women in particular, and perpetuates stereotypes of the male in search of gratification and the female in search of protection (Fine 1988). It may be extremely difficult for youth to be receptive to instruction that treats sexual decision making as only an informational, biological, social, moral, or cognitive process. They may also be unable to relate to a teacher who employs these approaches. Such approaches are not congruent with the teens' actual experience (Boxer et al. 1989).

We know that a sense of sexuality is informed by peers, culture, religion, and history; it is also informed by gender and racial relations of power (Fine 1988). If sex education does not explore both the joys and dangers of sexuality, there will be little opportunity for discussions beyond those constructed around male-centered definitions of heterosexuality. A discourse in which women have a voice—a discourse of desire—would be informed and generated out of their own socially constructed meanings.

Researchers have documented the negative correlation between teenagers' sex-negative attitudes and contraceptive use. Investigation of teenagers' contraceptive behavior indicates that individuals who feel either guilty or negative about their sexuality are less likely both to seek and to retain contraceptive information; they are also less likely to use contraceptives when sexually active than those who do not feel anxious and express positive feelings about sex (Schwartz 1973; Fisher et al. 1979). In other words, if teens believe sexual involvement is wrong, they are likely to deny responsibility for contraception, although they may engage, nonetheless, in sexual behavior.

Kirby has concluded that less than 10 percent of all public school students are exposed to what might be considered comprehensive sex education courses. The national evaluation of sex education programs conducted by Kirby and his associates (Kirby et al. 1979; Kirby 1983, 1984, 1985; see also Stout and Rivara 1989) indicates that most sex education courses increase knowledge. They generally have no statistically significant effect, however, on participants' (1) attitudes toward many sexually related topics, (2) patterns of communication with partners or parents about sex or birth control, (3) frequency of sexual intercourse, and (4) utilization of different methods of birth control. The only programs that had a clear influence on behavior were those that provided a directly relevant experiential component (for a review, see Boxer et al. 1989). For example, a parent-child workshop that actually initiated communication between parents and their children about sexuality produced improved communication. Similarly, when a health clinic was included in a high school's educational intervention program, the use of birth control increased, and births to teens were reduced. We do know that sex education in the public school can increase contraceptive knowledge and use.

It would, of course, be naive to expect a small number of hours devoted to sex education to be comprehensively effective.

However, recent research on school-based health clinics is quite promising (Edwards et al. 1980). Zabin and colleagues (Zabin et al. 1986) found that school-based health clinics that made referrals and dispensed contraceptives noted an increase in the percentage of virgin females visiting the clinic as well as an increase in contraceptive use. They also found a significant reduction in pregnancy rates. Eventually a substantial percentage of males visited the target clinic. Although counterintuitive, research has found that schools in which clinics dispensed contraceptives showed a substantial postponement of first experience of heterosexual intercourse among high school students and an increase in the proportion of young women visiting the clinic prior to first intercourse. The presence of such services may, then, enhance the females' sense of control and assure them that they are responsible and entitled to make their own decisions rather than being influenced by male pressures or prescriptions to control their sexuality.

As an example, Project Redirection (Polit et al. 1985) offers evidence of prevention of further pregnancy in a comprehensive vocational training and community-based mentor project for teen mothers and mothers-to-be in disadvantaged circumstances. The data indicate, however, that sustained positive outcomes cannot be expected when programs are withdrawn and participants must once again face their constricted life options.

Caution must be taken, however, not to revert to a "blame the victim" ideology. Attempting to intervene only among persons rather than social structures is not likely to succeed. Repeated motherhood may function as the only source of competence and hope for some young women without attractive life options. Socioeconomic conditions therefore directly contribute to sustaining teen pregnancy and birthrates. Sex education in the schools is a false panacea, but by providing meaningful education, counseling, and contraception as well as vocational opportunities, public schools can play a critical role in the sociosexual development of adolescents.

AIDS has, of course, changed the cultural significance of sexuality for everyone, in or out of school. Although adolescents are currently a very small proportion of those who have been diagnosed as having AIDS (Brooks-Gunn et al. 1988; Hein 1989), the risks for sexually active teens are increasing. AIDS has been a two-edged sword: It has somewhat increased the acceptability of discussions of sexuality in the public domain, but the impediments to adequate AIDS education remain serious and are similar to those regarding adolescent sexuality in general. For example, although AIDS education is now mandatory in Illinois, its implementation has been a slow process. Often the approach is piecemeal, left to the discretion of individual teachers, who themselves may have many unanswered questions about what to teach and how. On the other hand, outside the schools, alarm about AIDS has led to many innovative programs for youth that bluntly address sexuality, AIDS/HIV and ways to be protected from it. Recent studies demonstrate that teenagers have many misconceptions about the illness, including a sense of invulnverability, in part because of the cultural belief that AIDS is a gay illness (Brown et al. 1989; Center for Disease Control 1990; Hingson 1990).

A last word about adolescent sexuality—it is difficult to study. Ironically, it is more acceptable to school administrators, public officials, and parents for researchers to study teen pregnancy than adolescent sexuality. It is also difficult, as many of us well know, to study pubertal development. These cultural barriers also impede our ability to design effective interventions that take into account a developmental perspective on adolescent sexuality.

Adolescent Parenting and Life-Course Transitions

Developmentally, adolescents are in the process of constructing a set of future expectations of the life course yet to be. Other authors in this volume have pointed out how a baby may help create and sustain a sense of future for adolescent women with few life options. During late adolescence, school, work, and family-related decisions appear to be interwoven and thereby make late adolescence a time when there is often a pileup of role changes. The restructuring of personal expectations and anticipations for the future life course is a daunting developmental task for youth. Thus, enlarging opportunities for enhanced life options may help reduce the rate of unintended pregnancy among teens. When they are equipped with adequate vocational skills, a sense of self-worth, and psychosocial competence, their attitudes toward pregnancy may change.

Part of the problem posed by adolescent parenthood derives from disruption of a sequence that in our society assumes graduating from high school, entering the work force, marrying, and becoming a parent. Cohler (in press) has suggested that adolescent parenthood has been too often understood as a unique social problem rather than as one instance of problems of sequence and timing across the life course. Early off-time parenthood may be regarded as an accelerated role transition that represents one variation in the process of transition to parenthood, just as late off-time first parenthood may be regarded as an example of delayed role transition.

Although there are many variations in sequencing (Hogan 1982*b*), and there may be catch-up in terms of desirable adult outcomes (Furstenberg et al. this volume), role transitions that are off-time/off-sequence interfere with such later events as advancement at work or provision of economic support for family members among households headed by adolescent single mothers. In contrast to the late off-time assumption of the parental role, early off-time parenthood poses problems in finding role colleagues with whom to share this transition, lessens opportunity for anticipatory socialization into the parental role apart from the specific details of child care, and disrupts sequencing of expectable life course events. Of all early off-time life changes, the transition to parenthood during the mid-adolescent years is probably the most disruptive for a new parent and the larger family unit.

Findings to date about the transition to parenthood among adolescents leave many questions unanswered. As noted by Furstenberg, Brooks-Gunn, and Morgan (1987), social change over the last twenty years means that many studies must be replicated with new cohorts of adolescent parents. Much of the existing research has been concerned primarily with structural characteristics. The psychosocial interior of the family is seldom explored in this research; little information is available about relations among the new mother, her own parents, and the baby's father, or the mother's tie to the child. Existing data suggest that although adolescent mothers may be less well informed than their older counterparts about child care, they do not differ in terms of warmth and overall quality of care (Furstenberg 1976), nor do their infants show adverse developmental patterns beyond the increased risk so often documented among infants born into families living in poverty (Furstenberg et al., this volume).

Since the Enlightenment, our culture has come to believe that childhood is a time of frailty and that parental failures in providing optimal caregiving, particularly on the part of mothers, are largely responsible for variations seen among the children in later life (Ariès 1962). A child's maturation and development are understood in our society as determined largely by parental care. We do know now, of course, that children make a contribution to their own development. Socialization from parent to child and from child to parent is a reciprocal process. This process has barely been examined with regard to adolescent mothers and their children.

Understanding this process has particular implications for the adolescents' development, since one of the problems associated with adolescent entrance into parenthood is that the role of parent, typically associated with attainment of adult status, conflicts with shared definitions of the adolescents as still dependent and not yet adult. Changes in this role status affect the ways in which interdependencies between adolescents and their parents are negotiated. Burton (1990) and others have highlighted ways in which the birth of a child to an adolescent affects the adolescent's family, and in particular the adolescent's mother. These developmental reciprocities have, however, been little studied. And most important here, how parent-adolescent bonds are affected and restructured has been studied even less, although understanding their implications for adult functioning seems critical.

A strong cultural ideal portrays adolescence as the time when enduring separations are initiated between parents and children (Greene and Boxer 1986). Writers frequently describe the task of young adulthood as separation from the family and the successful assumption of new, autonomous social roles. At the psychological level, Blos (1962) characterizes adolescence and young adulthood as part of a second individuation process. At the social level, this perspective is complemented by the use of extrafamilial markers (marriage, establishing an independent household, or parenthood) to index both the degree and timeliness with which the young adult has effected this transition.

However, an increasing corpus of research points to the maintenance of parent-child bonds over the life course (see, e.g., Troll and Bengtson 1982). Despite differences in maturational levels, geographic propinquity, gender, and socioeconomic mobility, as well as possibly confounding effects of cultural change and peer interaction, parent-child solidarity consistently appears to represent an important interpersonal bond in contemporary American culture. Our cultural view of adolescents as needing to become totally autonomous is an ideal rarely achieved. Rather, it appears that what is achieved is not familial autonomy but familial interdependence, a state of differentiation rather than separation, in which the maintenance of parental bonds and independent functioning are dual achievements. The question is thus not one of separation or its timeliness but the processes by which the family's interdependence is renegotiated over successive mutual transitions (Greene and Boxer 1986).

The transition to adulthood heralds, then, a renegotiation of autonomy and dependency. Typically, role changes outside of the family, such as marriage or childbirth, affect parent and child in restructuring their interactions consequent to the child's new social status. My colleague Anita Greene and I (Greene and Boxer 1986) have termed these boundary facilitators. For example, the new marital status of a young adult we interviewed in our transition study can be seen as an example of how an extrafamilial event facilitated the development of new types of boundaries between parent and child. This young woman told us:

> My mother really treats me differently now. . . . Before she would want to know what I was doing, who I was with, you know . . . personal stuff. Now she starts to do it and she stops and says, "Oh, . . . you're a married woman, I can't say that anymore. You have your own life now." . . . Wasn't it my life before? . . . If I'd known getting married would give me this much weight, I'd have done it when I was twelve. [Greene and Boxer 1986: 141]

Another renegotiation strategy affecting a reorganization of bonds between parent and child we have termed boundary disruptors. These include dropping out of school, divorce, separation, and loss of employment. Such events provide both parents and children adaptive leverage in the differentiation process. In certain instances, this may be the only means through which a child is able to effect renegotiation in the family. Adolescent pregnancy is an example of this process. A child may venture beyond his or her situation within the family to achieve differentiation and recognition of adult status. A critical aspect of this transition is its acceptability to others in the family. We hope that future research on these transitions will enlighten us in understanding developmental reciprocities for parent, adolescent, and offspring as well.

Much of the study of adolescent parenthood has assumed, in common with other longitudinal developmental studies, that experience early in life has a single, unitary, continuous effect on later life. The life-span perspective presented here does not support that linear cause-and-effect model. The *timing* of entrance into expectable adult roles needs to be disaggregated, for purposes of investigation, from the *sequence* of entrance into those roles. Separating timing from sequence will enable us to understand further what factors contribute to achievement of successful transitions into the adult life course. It should also offer us a better picture of how the reciprocal socialization of the mother and baby intersects with the continuing intrafamilial role negotiations of mother and father with their own mothers and fathers.

NOTES

Preparation of this manuscript was facilitated by an institutional training grant from the National Institute of Mental Health (#5T32 MH14668-14) entitled "A Clinical Research Training Program in Adolescence."

[1] This does not obviate the need to quantify adolescent sexual behaviors and the frequency of their occurrence, or predictors of sexual behavior and sexual risk taking. However, researchers studying adolescent sexuality typically neglect specific behaviors (see also Brooks-Gunn and Furstenberg 1989), and, instead, focus on global outcomes such as "sexual behavior" in general, or sexual intercourse. These terms may be differentially interpreted by adolescents as signifying behaviors other than those intended by researchers (see Herdt and Boxer 1991).

DONNA L. FRANKLIN

4 Early Childbearing Patterns Among African Americans: A Socio-Historical Perspective

During the 1980s, analysts were concerned about a small group of African American families headed by women, concentrated in the inner cities, whose salient characteristics included persistent poverty and family formation patterns different from those of mainstream Americans. Numerous causal frameworks have emerged in the social science literature over time to explain the origin of these patterns, with much of the attention given to the higher rates of childbearing among African American adolescents than among white adolescents.

Birthrates among African American adolescents have historically been much higher than birthrates among whites. The current variance in the fertility rates between these two groups is viewed as problematic (Franklin 1988b). Social analysts are unclear what mixture of factors—sociological, environmental, and cultural—have historically driven these higher rates of adolescent parenthood among African Americans. More recently, sharp declines in postdelivery African American adolescent marriages and marital fertility rates have contributed to dramatic changes in family structure among African Americans.

It is the historical phenomenon of adolescent childbearing among African Americans, however, that will be the major focus of this chapter. Its objective is to review and provide a descriptive analysis of the social science literature that has addressed the issue of adolescent childbearing and related issues and to attempt to identify and organize competing explanations for them. These explanations have ranged from those that have focused on the moral and behavioral aspects of the problem to the more recent scholarship, represented by William Julius Wilson (1987) and Beatrix Hamburg (1986), which offers a comprehensive analysis of the problem most useful for public policy analysts.

This chapter is written from a developmental perspective that directs attention to the way that the African American family as a subsystem has been transformed over time by evolving social mores and to its interaction with societal institutions. Using the ideas that were first presented by Burgess (1926), who inaugurated the field of family relations, this approach focuses on changes that have taken place in the family as a subsystem and have shaped the family formation patterns found among poor African American families residing in inner-city communities today. Allen (1978) also developed a typology for evaluating theoretical and ideological approaches to the study of the black family that will be useful in providing a framework for critically evaluating the studies presented in this essay in its summary section.

The Institution of Slavery

Any discussion of black family formation patterns must begin with the institution of slavery. The roots of the African American family were planted in the mid and late eighteenth century, when slaves combined African and American cultural beliefs and practices into a distinctive African American system of family and kinship with its own rules of courtship, sexual behavior, and marriage. The courting and mating practices of African slaves and their early African American descendants have been little studied, so it is hard to describe how enslavement affected those practices. Yet historians seem to agree that slaves were operating under a different subculture than the slaveholders. Gutman holds: "much indirect evidence suggests a close relationship between the relatively early age of a slave woman at the birth of a first child, prenuptial intercourse, slave attachments to a family of origin and to enlarged slave kin networks, and the economic needs of slaveowners" (1976:75). The system of slavery put a high premium on females who, whether married or single, began early to bear children. For the owner, the birth of a slave child was economic in nature, while the same event was viewed by the slave as social and familial. Early childbearing and subsequent high fertility greatly increased a married or unmarried woman's value to her owner and thereby diminished the likelihood of her sale and physical separation from her family."

Mintz and Kellogg (1988) agree with Gutman that distinctive African American patterns of life, social codes, and social attitudes were also shaped by the economy of slavery. Even though marriages were illegal, slaves still celebrated marriages in religious ceremonies or in rites during which the couple would jump over a broomstick. And although slave masters sometimes even recognized marriage by declaring a holiday or giving the couple a separate cabin or gift, the vulnerability of these marriages was still quite apparent (Gutman 1976; Blassingame 1979). Masters could terminate slave unions and spouses had no legal rights. For two people contemplating marriage, one of the ways of increasing the probability that they would remain together was by beginning to have children early. In this way, their owners would have both economic and ethical reasons to allow them to remain together (Gutman 1976).

Sexual behavior among slaves followed a set of clearly defined standards that were not consistent with the prevailing norms of whites. The owner of a Georgia plantation described the standards that she believed slaves adhered to: "The Negroes had their own ideals of morality, and held to them very strictly; they did not consider it wrong for a girl to have a child before she married, but afterwards were extremely severe upon anything like infidelity on her part" (Litwack 1979:243). African American preachers vehemently opposed premarital intercourse, and churches imposed sanctions on offenders found guilty of fornication (Genovese 1974; Gutman 1976). Genovese (1974) is one of the few social scientists to point out that the extent of "fornication, illegitimacy and adultery" among "lower class whites" also remains "problematical" and that there is no reason to believe that "it was one whit less than among the slaves" (466).

Slave society was a subculture in which the norms about marriage and the family were different from the general societal norms. The institution of slavery further reinforced the differences. Under slave law, African American men, women, and children were regarded as individual units of property, and marriage between slaves was not legally recognized. The concept of legitimacy did not apply to African Americans during the period of slavery. Children belonged to their master, who was viewed as having custody of all his slaves, adults and children alike. This fact rendered early childbearing functional for the slaveholders.

The Effects of
Changing Migration Patterns

After Emancipation, between 1870 and 1910, an average of 6,700 Southern blacks moved North annually. From 1916 to 1921, an estimated half a million blacks headed North, most of them from the Deep South (Johnson and Campbell 1981). Two recently published books have also chronicled the movement from the Deep South to northern industrial centers (Grossman 1989; Lemann 1991). Before this more recent interest in migration patterns among blacks, scholars had noted that changes in the residential patterns of African Americans in the South were altering their family structure. The same scholars did not agree, however, in interpreting how these shifting migration patterns were influencing black family life.

When Woofter (1971 [1920]) studied 742 African American women with children in Athens, Georgia, he found that 4 percent were single or never married, 16 percent were widowed, 7 percent were separated, and 73 percent were living with a husband. When he compared white and black females fifteen years old and over, he found 26.6 percent of the blacks were single and 30.1 percent of the whites. He attributed these differences to earlier marriages among African American women.[1]

Woofter was one of the first social scientists to report on the effects of the migration on the African American family. Young women and men furnished the majority of migrants from the Black Belt. Young African American men, in Woofter's view, were moving to agricultural areas for work, while the young women were moving to areas where there were more domestic service opportunities. The different migratory patterns of males and females were causing sex ratio imbalances and changes in family structure. These alterations contributed to the "disorganization" of the African American family. Woofter expressed concern that large numbers of females without spouses were rearing children.

Johnson (1934) provided a more in-depth look at the family formation patterns found among rural blacks living in the South when he studied 600 African American families living in Alabama. He described these families as experiencing a "great deal of cultural isolation." He also noted that the sex ratio was imbalanced and observed a "large number of women heads of families." Like Woofter, Johnson found earlier marriages, higher fertility rates, and larger families among African American women as compared to whites. Johnson noted that an interest in children and large families might have been a carryover from the period of slavery when the "social status among Negro slave women was in an important measure based upon their breeding power" (58).

Johnson went further than Woofter, however, when he provided a context for evaulating the differences between urban and rural African Americans living in the South. In rural areas, according to Johnson, the family as an organization was the most efficient unit for raising cotton and food. Early marriages were discouraged because the economic unit of the family was upset when a young person married and left home. Therefore, when young couples married, they were expected to live in and become part of the household of the parents. Johnson discussed the problems that were created by the postponement of marriage in rural areas:

> The active passions of youth and late adolescence are present but without the usual formal social restraints. Social behavior rooted in this situation, even when its consequences are understood, is lightly censured or excused entirely. . . . When pregnancy follows, pressure is not strong enough to compel the father either to marry the mother or to support the child. The girl does not lose status, perceptibly, nor are her chances for marrying seriously threatened. . . . There is, in a sense, no such thing as illegitimacy in this community. [1934:49]

Of the 612 families Johnson studied, 12 mothers with children were never married, 105 were widowed, and 52 were married but separated. He also noted that a number of women, now married, had had a child before marriage. While Johnson never used the term "social class" to describe the differences between rural and urban blacks, the rural blacks he describes were poor blacks working as sharecroppers and living under the hegemony of the landowner. Johnson's descriptions of family formation patterns among blacks make distinctions between the behavioral patterns found among blacks based on different social conditions. (See also Dollard 1937; Davis et al. 1941.)

Elaborating further on some of Johnson's observations regarding rural life in the South, E. Franklin Frazier built on the idea of class as culture and predicted that social norms that were relatively benign in the closely knit rural South would have disastrous consequences as blacks migrated to Northern cities:

> It is impossible to draw any conclusion from available statistics concerning either the volume or trend of illegitimacy among Negroes . . . illegitimacy is from five to ten times as high among Negroes as among whites. . . . Undoubtedly, much of the illegitimacy issues from social disorganization and results in personal demoralization. . . . During the course of their migration to the city, family ties are broken, and the restraints which once held in check immoral sex conduct lose

their force. Hence at the same time that simple rural families are losing their internal cohesion, they are being freed from the controlling force of public opinion and communal institutions. [1966:259, 265, 267]

We have found different explanations for higher rates of unmarried motherhood and single-parent households among African Americans when compared to whites. Woofter blamed the migration patterns for creating imbalances in gender ratios of African American men to women because males had to look in different regions or areas for the kind of work they were seeking. Johnson, on the other hand, viewed two distinct cultures as existing in the rural and urban areas and saw the economic exigencies of the sharecropping system as creating differential norms with respect to courtship, childbearing, and marriage. Both Woofter and Johnson indicated that African American women were marrying earlier and having more children than white women and noted that there was a great deal of sexual activity before marriage. The family formation patterns found among poor African Americans were not traced to slavery by these analysts, however, even though Johnson noted that an interest in children and large families may have been a carryover from slavery. Neither Johnson nor Woofter reported large numbers of families headed by never-married women. It seems clear from their descriptions that a number of children were born to women before marriage, but most of these women eventually married the father of their children. It was Frazier (1966) who predicted that these family formation patterns would prove problematic as African Americans migrated North.

The Baby-Boom Years

During the early 1940s, we find one of the first references to increases in birthrates among unmarried women. Gunnar Myrdal, in his classic *American Dilemma,* noted that there was an "extremely high illegitimacy rate among Negroes" (1944:177). When Myrdal compared white and black birthrates for the unmarried, he found that in 1936 the rates for African Americans were 16.2 percent, for whites, 2.0 percent. He expressed concern about the social handicaps to which these black children would be subjected:

Even if the [child] has a good mother, she cannot give him the proper care since she must usually earn her own living and cannot afford to place him under proper supervision. The absence of a father is detrimental to the development of a child's personality. . . . The unwed mother tends—although there are many exceptions—to have looser morals and lower standards, and in this respect does not provide the proper milieu for her child. It would be better for society in general and for the mother if she had no child. [178]

Myrdal thus elaborates on Frazier's concerns about the social disadvantages that the child born out of wedlock will face in society, and—like Frazier—offers no data whatsoever to support his supposition. He proceeds further with his moralistic denigration of the unwed mother and the consequences that will accrue to her child, who suffers because of her inability to parent and the absence of the father. This is the first time that we see the emergence of a perspective that does not attempt to place the occurrence of the births within any particular subcultural context. Myrdal does not discuss social and economic factors in an effort to explain changes in black family structure.

One year later, Drake and Cayton (1945) published their seminal study of the black community in Chicago and elaborated on the structural features of the black family. In their discussion of the increasing disorganization of the low-income family, they attributed changes in the family structure to the "high rates of desertion, illegitimacy, and divorce as well as a great deal of violent conflict in the lower-class household." The authors viewed black men as lacking economic opportunity, which then contributed to the shifting of responsibility to the women in these households, who "almost always hold the purse strings." They further elaborated the effect this had on the black men, who, insecure in their economic power, "tend to exalt their sexual prowess" (1945:582).

Drake and Cayton also observed that greater numbers of children were being born to families without fathers living in the household. They described the unwed mothers as being members of the lower class who "had been in the city less than five years." In their view, "such an 'accident' rarely [happened] to girls in other social classes, or even to lower-class girls wise in the way of the city." They further asserted that the adjustment to being an unwed mother was made in one of the following ways. (1) In two-parent families, the daughter could live with her parents and contribute to the support of her family. (2) In mother-only families, the daughter could work while the grandmother cared for the child; or if no work was available "relief provided for the family unit." (3) She could set up an independent household and depend on "relief" for support. Or (4) she could "find a 'boyfriend' to support herself and [her] child" (1945:590). Drake and Cayton also noted, as had others who preceded them, that the "lower-class does not make a grave social or moral issue of illegitimacy" (593).

Their view is somewhat consistent with Frazier's that the most recent immigrants to the industrial North were the most vulnerable to out-of-wedlock pregnancy, but they did not trace, as he did, the behavioral patterns to the rural South. Theirs is the first description we have, however, of the economic plight of the black male in the urban North and its effect on family stability, the black male's self-image, and the tension created between black males and females.

For the first time, we see the concept of family "disorganization" tied to the shifts in women's occupational status. World War II brought dramatic improvements in the working lives of black women, according to Kessler-Harris (1982). Approximately 20 percent of those who had been domestic servants moved into the jobs white women vacated when they moved into factory work. The combined effect of the Fair Employment Practices Commission, created in July 1941, union pressure, and demonstrations on the part of black women resulted in a 15 percent drop in domestic work; the number of black women in clerical sales, and even of black women professional workers, increased substantially.

Drake and Cayton (1945) noted the increase in family "disorganization" and attributed it to men's joining the armed forces and women's entering the work force in increasing numbers. It seems ironic that the war would bring blacks out of economic depression and simultaneously create more problems for the black family. Drake and Cayton document the changing agendas during this period, changes that would profoundly affect the future of the black family.

The Effect of the Northern Ghetto

By the 1950s, it was becoming clear that the dynamics of discrimination in employment and housing in the industrial North were devastating its black residents. For example, the favorable educational position of blacks compared to the new immigrants had declined; black male unemployment rates were two or three times higher than those of foreign-born whites; black women's joblessness rates were three to four times greater than those of foreign-born whites (Lieberson 1980). From 1890 to 1950, marriage rates among blacks had exceeded those of whites, but after 1950 black marriage rates fell below white rates and continued to decline (Engerman 1977).

After 1950, census statistics reflect that the numbers of blacks in urban areas were increasing and the numbers of whites were decreasing as they moved to the suburbs, a trend that continues to the present. These shifts in population contributed to the changes in housing and neighborhood patterns in Northern cities and subsequently to the creation and the persistence of the black urban slum. In *Beyond the Melting Pot,* Glazer and Moynihan described these blighted areas:

The slums now contain the very large families that are not eligible for public housing because they would overcrowd it; the families that have been ejected from the projects (or were never admitted) for being antisocial; those who have either recently arrived in the city and hardly adapted to urban life, or those who may have been here a long time but never adapted; as well as the dope peddlers and users, the sex perverts and criminals, the pimps and prostitutes whom the managers reject or eject to protect the population. All these are now concentrated in the slums that ring the projects, and areas that were perhaps just barely tolerable before the impact of the projects are now quite intolerable. [1963:63–64]

In the mid-1960s, Kenneth Clark wrote about his experiences in working with youth in Harlem. Some of the key elements found in Frazier's work, namely, the value-laden and moralistic commentary, were absent in Clark's writings, conceived as a study of disorganization and different attitudes toward sex. Clark viewed sex in the middle class as mainly symbolic and used to attain status, while for the poor it was an end in itself. In his view it fulfilled emotional needs for affection and self-esteem and carried no expectation of long-term obligation between partners. He attempted to explain higher rates of out-of-wedlock births among young black women, which he viewed as carrying a meaning different for poor blacks from the mainstream's evaluation: "In the ghetto, the meaning of the illegitimate child is not the ultimate disgrace. There is not the demand for abortion or surrender of the child that one finds in more privileged communities. The child is proof of womanhood, something of her own to have" (1967:72). Clark felt these social behaviors were attempts to meet basic human needs in an environment that allowed few opportunities for fulfillment. In this analysis, Clark took the argument to a new level by focusing on the foundation values and moved the focus away from the topic of sexual activity that had dominated some of the earlier writings to highlight instead attitudes underlying sexual behavior.

Also in the mid-60s Rainwater (1966) observed a "subculture" among the black low-income residents of a public housing project in St. Louis that was distinct from middle-class norms and mores. The risks of pregnancy, as he reported, were far outweighed by the immediate gratification of the need for self-esteem and love provided by the sexual relationship. Rainwater made one major point of departure from the earlier tradition, however: he noted that, even with a separate behavioral subculture, the poor hold the same ideal norms and values as the middle class. When circumstances militate against their achieving these ideal standards of behavior, however, the poor develop an adaptive set of alternative norms that guide their social behavior.

The effect of the out-migration from the rural South to the industrial North, and the unforeseen factors associated with it, is most clearly observed in the precipitous increase in black adolescent birthrates. From 1940 to 1972, the number of births to unmarried black adolescents ages fifteen to nineteen doubled; by 1977 the rate was more than six times that for white adolescents (U.S. Commission on Civil Rights 1983). Teenage mothers constituted a greater proportion of single mothers than ever before in both the black and white community. And when Moynihan (1965) analyzed the changing trends in welfare from 1948 to 1961, he found that black families accounted for two-thirds of the increases in the Aid to Dependent Children program. Moynihan did not explore the relationships between escalating adolescent births and increased dependency on ADC, however, but instead quoted Frazier extensively and described a lower-class "subculture" characterized by "matriarchy," emasculated males, educational failure, delinquency, crime, and drug addiction.

In the 1960s, for the first time in American history, a large proportion of young people from their teens into their twenties developed a separate existence, relatively free of the demands of adulthood and more independent of parental supervision than that of children in previous generations. This youth culture was tied together by a common orientation: alienation from adult roles and values (Keniston 1965). One of the behaviors that proliferated in this youth culture was an early initiation into sexual activity, and most of this activity occurred outside of marriage. While black youths are often overlooked in these analyses of youth culture, they were not exempt from these shifts in sexual and marital mores.

For example, one of the changes we see between 1960 and 1970 is the declining marriage rates among both black and white adolescent parents. Adolescent birthrates and marriage statistics in Illinois are an example. Before 1960, less than 14 percent of the children born to black adolescents were born to women unmarried at the time of the child's birth. By 1970 that proportion had risen to 40 percent, and by 1983 the figure had climbed to 66 percent. The increases for whites are comparable, although somewhat lower. Testa and Lawlor, discussing these striking trends, assert "today virtually no black teenage mothers are married at the time of delivery" (1985:30).

Social policymakers have been particularly alarmed by the declining marriage rates among black women and the fact that black families were increasingly headed by never-married women rather than by divorced, widowed, or separated women (Darity and Myers 1984; McLanahan and Garfinkel 1989). Some recent studies have related these changes to a declining ratio of men to women in the black community, reflecting some combination of males' higher rates of mortality, incarceration, and homelessness (Darity and Myers 1984; Center for the Study of Social Policy 1984; Wilson 1987). Given these changes, many of the resulting mother-only households are financially vulnerable.

In their analysis of black urban life, Nathan Glazer and Daniel Patrick Moynihan described life in the urban ghettos:

Broken homes and illegitimacy do not necessarily mean poor upbringing and emotional problems. But they mean it more often when the mother is forced to work (as the Negro mother so often is), when the father is incapable of contributing to support (as the Negro father so often is), when fathers and mothers refuse to accept responsibility for and resent their children, as Negro parents, overwhelmed by difficulties, so often do, and when the family situation . . . is left vague and ambiguous (as it so often is in Negro families). [1963:50]

Two years following the publication of this book, a confidential report was released by the federal government, also written by Moynihan (1965). This report brought the plight of the black family to the public's attention. The breakdown of the black family, in Moynihan's view, had led to sharp increases in welfare dependency, delinquency, illegitimacy, unemployment, drug addiction, and failure in school. Moynihan attributed the instability of the black family to the effects of slavery and of the structural changes, such as rapid urbanization and years of severe unemployment, that had undermined the role of the black man in the family.

Early Childbearing as an
Alternative Life-Course Strategy

An approach to the study of family relations that was inaugurated by Burgess (1926) asserts that people are changed by changing families and that families are changed by the changing behavior and the developmental course of members. In his essay, "The Family as a Unit of Interacting Personalities" (1926), he makes the point that by person or personality he refers to the social self with the roles and expectations of others it has internalized. These expectations, in Burgess's view, are constantly being challenged and reshaped by evolving social mores. They have important implications when applied to the changes in family life that have emerged over time among African Americans living in poverty.

Building on this basic idea, Lewis (1966a) developed the concept of the "culture of poverty" to describe how the effects of poverty were being transmitted intergenerationally in the poor families he studied in Puerto Rico. Lewis was something of a socialist and saw this culture as an inescapable by-product of competitive capitalism. The "culture" issue was politicized in the late 1960s, however, and used by conservatives to blame the individuals living in poverty and thereby erode support for social reforms. Working from a more recent development of the concept of social isolation and consistent with the principles set forth by Burgess, Wilson (1987) proffered a thesis asserting greater responsiveness of behavior to variations in objective social constraints and opportunities.

Other more recent attempts by social scientists have addressed the questions that Lewis was grappling with in the 1960s. First, are children who grow up in families headed by single women who bore children during their adolescent years more vulnerable to persistent poverty? And second, if they are, how is that poverty transmitted from one generation to the next? The literature that attempts to address these questions is quite extensive, and the answers are not definitive. (See Ross and Sawhill 1975; Shinn 1978; Hetherington et al. 1983; Aponte 1988; and Franklin 1988a,b for reviews of this literature.) Those who have evaluated income data agree that offspring who live in families with more education and two parents present have higher rates of employment and consistently higher standards of living (Featherman and Hauser 1978; Hill et al. 1985; McLanahan 1986). And studies that have evaluated the family formation patterns of the offspring from single-parent families have found that these children are more likely either to marry early or to have children early. This pattern is even more pronounced among low-income families (Bumpass and Sweet 1972; Heiss 1972; McLanahan and Bumpass 1986).

Campbell (1968) was one of the first social scientists to identify the adverse effects of early childbearing on the lives of adolescent mothers. Numerous studies have since confirmed Campbell's prognosis for poorer socioeconomic outcomes for adolescent mothers. These studies have found that women who give birth during the teenage years complete fewer years of schooling, hold lower-paying jobs, and experience more marital instability than adolescents who delay childbearing until their adult years (Furstenberg 1976; Card and Wise 1978; Hofferth and Moore 1979; Kellam et al. 1982; Marini 1984; O'Connell and Rogers 1984).

In research conducted more recently, however, the role of early child-bearing in predicting educational and employment outcomes is less clear, and this has been puzzling to social scientists. For example, one of the few longitudinal studies found that a large number of adolescent mothers in the study sample were able to finish their high school education, find employment, and move away from welfare dependency (Furstenberg et al. 1987). Another study found that the role of early childbearing in ending schooling early is much less clear when comparisons are drawn between women who were teenagers when they bore children and women in similar income categories who delayed childbearing until they were adults (Upchurch and McCarthy 1990).

How do we explain these seemingly disparate findings? Duncan and Hoffman (1991) tackled this question in "Teenage Underclass Behavior and Subsequent Poverty: Have the Rules Changed?" They conducted an analysis by using two sources, Panel Survey of Income Dynamics and census data, to describe the trends in fertility and schooling among adolescents since the late 1960s. They found that, although there was an increase in schooling of white and black teenagers and little change in the incidence of out-of-wedlock births, "the labor market involvement of black women who had either dropped out of high school or had an out-of-wedlock birth had declined by the 1980s, while their reliance on AFDC had become much greater" (15). These authors conclude that "one rule does appear to have changed . . . that schooling and delayed childbearing are sufficient conditions for most women to avoid poverty as adults. Our evidence does not tell us whether this rule continues to hold for the minority of women living in concentrated poverty areas of our nation's cities." Duncan and Hoffman close by stating that "the deteriorating opportunities may be crucial in explaining the extraordinarily high rates of teen births and welfare dependence in some of our nation's cities" (29).

A complementary explanation of the changes found in the above study has been set forth by Hamburg (1986), who noted that family formation patterns among black women in poor urban communities are reflecting an "alternative life course strategy" rather than a nonnormative life event. She asserts further that these patterns may be a response to compelling developmental, social, and economic factors unique to the mother's subculture. Hamburg identifies a subculture more comprehensively than earlier analyses that focused on either the sexual activities or the value structure as causal factors. Burton's (1990) three-year exploratory study of adolescent childbearing in twenty low-income multigenerational black families further documents the family formation patterns of these women as having four distinct characteristics: (1) an accelerated family timetable; (2) separation of reproduction and marriage; (3) an age-condensed generational family structure; and (4) a grandparental child-rearing system. Although Burton's qualitative research strategy did not involve the use of a representative sample of black families, her in-depth analysis does enhance our understanding of why childbearing during the adolescent years is no longer the strongest predictor of the negative sequelae associated with early transition to the parenting role.

Summary

This chapter has chronicled the explanatory frameworks that have emerged in the literature during different historical periods to explain family formation patterns among blacks. What are the implications of this history? Allen's (1978) concepts of cultural equivalence, cultural deviance, and cultural variance provide a typology for considering some of the studies reported here. The *equivalence* approach emphasizes the features that black families have in common with white families; the *deviance* approach points to qualities that distinguish blacks from whites; and the *variance* approach calls for contextually relevant interpretations of black family life.

This chapter was written from a developmental perspective and has focused attention on the change in African American family formation patterns over time by describing the interplay of the family as a subsystem with other institutions in society. It begins by describing the subculture that existed during slavery and cites studies that have traced these early childbearing patterns to slavery and have endeavored to explain the persistence of these patterns even after slavery was abolished. Some of these studies were narrowly focused on the sexual or moral conduct or both of blacks that was behind these different family formation patterns. Terms like "social disorganization" and "social pathology" were used to describe these different American sharecropping families in the Deep South. The cultural equivalent and cultural deviant approaches delineated by Walter Allen are most clearly reflected in the works of both E. Franklin Frazier and Charles S. Johnson, who asserted that middle-income blacks were the cultural equivalent of whites and that low-income blacks were culturally deviant from whites and middle-class blacks.

One example of an application of the cultural equivalent and cultural deviant approaches can be found in an analysis set forth by Frazier in his seminal study of blacks in the city of Chicago. Frazier demonstrated that, as blacks moved from the poverty-stricken inner cities where the new immigrants generally settled to the periphery where the more acculturated blacks resided, there was a decrease in factors associated with "social disorganization." He made specific reference to factors such as "illegitimacy and female-headed households." In the introduction of Frazier's 1939 book, Ernest Burgess noted that this finding demonstrated rather conclusively that black family life varied almost as widely as white family life.

When blacks started to migrate North, these explanatory approaches were gradually expanded with an emphasis that shifted the focus to the breakdown in the socialization process. Frazier is generally credited with initiating this approach in the literature, which climaxed with the Moynihan report. This approach generally blames mother-only families for perpetuating behaviors that do not conform to societal norms. Vitriolic attacks were directed at Moynihan, a self-anointed liberal, by black scholars and politicians who challenged his analysis. They noted that his argument, following in the tradition of Frazier and Johnson, was equating blacks' nonconformity to middle-class values with instability and disorganization. Clark and Rainwater are credited with an approach at this same time that placed an emphasis on different values held by residents of lower-income communities without the moral overtones that had characterized the earlier analyses.

Less frequently social scientists explain early childbearing among blacks as demonstrating how social problems are interactively shaped by both the group's behavioral norms and changing social forces. The distinctive element here is the contextual component; it is what Allen refers to as the cultural variant approach. It is finally this key concept that emerges to link the multiple determinants of the problem—as reflected in the Hamburg formulation and in the writings of William J. Wilson, Linda Burton, and others. This more comprehensive analysis of the problem will advance discussion toward alternative ways of addressing current social and economic arrangements to improve conditions for these families. With this in mind, we should understand more clearly why our panoply of interventions with these families—ahistorical and narrowly focused—have been inappropriate. A public policy directed at poor black mothers' needs must carefully consider the group's distinct history within the American societal context, both when conceptualizing its problems and when proposing policy solutions.

NOTE

1. In a later study Woofter (1930) observed the family formation patterns among young black Sea Islanders and noted that a significant percentage of births occurred regularly before marriage but added that many couples married afterward, so the problem was not as great as birth statistics might indicate. Woofter attributed these births to inadequate knowledge of contraception and did not focus on the moral issues raised by other authors during that period.

JEWELLE TAYLOR GIBBS

5 The Social Context of Teenage Pregnancy and Parenting in the Black Community: Implications for Public Policy

The proliferation of literature on adolescent pregnancy mirrors its significance as a social problem and its complexity as a behavioral phenomenon. Although the literature encompasses a diverse range of ethnographic, demographic, clinical, and empirical investigations, these studies have traditionally focused on female adolescents (Furstenberg et al. 1981; Zelnik et al. 1983; Chilman 1983). Only in recent years have researchers discovered an obvious connection between the sexual behaviors, pregnancy, and parenting experiences of female adolescents and the sexual behaviors, social experiences, and marital attitudes of their male partners (Clark et al. 1984; Sander and Rosen 1987; Robinson 1988). Although this connection itself may be obvious, the relation among these factors appears to be extremely complex and continues to present challenges to social science researchers and to provoke controversy among social policy planners.

Nowhere is the debate over the most effective research strategy or the most appropriate social policy options more intense than on the topic of out-of-wedlock pregnancy among black adolescent females. Many hypotheses have been advanced to explain the high rates of pregnancy and subsequent birthrates among unwed black teenagers. In an excellent review article, Franklin (1988*b*) summarized these hypotheses using an ecological framework that includes individual, family, sociocultural, and social structural dimensions.

This chapter has two goals: (1) to examine the effect of these four interrelated dimensions on the sexual behaviors, pregnancy, and parenting experiences of black adolescent females, with a special focus on the contribution of young black males to these behaviors and experiences; and (2) to propose policies that would modify significant aspects of the social structural dimension impinging on the lives of black youth so that, in turn, their sociocultural context would eventually reinforce a new set of sexual attitudes, behaviors, and experiences.

Scope of the Problem

A brief review of statistics on teenage pregnancy indicates the scope of the problem. In 1989, black females accounted for 15.8 percent of the adolescent female population but were responsible for 30.4 percent of all teenage births. By age eighteen, 26 percent of black females have given birth, and 40 percent have a child before age twenty (Children's Defense Fund 1988). Black teenagers also account for 39 percent of all repeat births to adolescent mothers. Black teenage birthrates are twice as high as white rates, and black teenage mothers are 60 percent more likely than their white counterparts to be unmarried (92% vs. 56%) (National Center for Health Statistics 1991). While adolescent birthrates consistently dropped among single black females between 1960 and 1983, there were steady increases among single white teenagers, suggesting the effect of broader social and economic forces on out-of-wedlock childbearing and family formation (Children's Defense Fund 1988). Between 1983 and 1989, however, the birthrate of black females aged fifteen to nineteen increased 20 percent, while the birthrate for white adolescent females increased only 8.4 percent during the same six-year period (National Center for Health Statistics 1991). This difference in birthrates between black and white females cannot be explained solely in terms of rates of sexual activity but appears to be the result of different patterns of sexual behaviors, contraceptive use, and childbearing decisions.

Adolescent pregnancy is a problem for the mother and her infant, physically, psychologically, and socially. Short-term follow-up studies of teenage parents have generally painted a portrait of less than optimal consequences of early childbearing (Furstenberg et al. 1981; Chilman 1983; O'Connell and Rogers 1984). More recent research, however, suggests a range of outcomes mediated by a complex set of factors including differential resources, motivational levels, intervention programs, career experiences, and marital decisions (Geronimus 1987; Upchurch and McCarthy 1990; Luker 1991). In comparing outcomes in a seventeen-year follow-up of their Baltimore sample with data from several national samples, Furstenberg and his colleagues found that early childbearers had more negative social and economic outcomes than late childbearers, but differences between these groups were fewer and less dramatic than expected, especially with respect to family size and long-term welfare dependency (Furstenberg et al. 1987).

Because of the less than optimal consequences for the majority of teenage mothers, major efforts have been directed toward preventing the first pregnancy of those adolescent girls considered to be at high risk for parenthood. Secondary prevention efforts have focused on early intervention with adolescent mothers to improve their parenting skills and to enhance their life options through education or employment training programs. But these efforts have not been uniformly successful, and, in fact, some follow-up studies have shown disappointing results (Polit and Kahn 1985; Weatherley et al. 1986). Perhaps it is time to step back from the evaluation of these specific programs and to ask a much broader set of questions. (1) How could the design and implementation of programs incorporate an adequate understanding of the ecological and sociocultural context in which adolescent pregnancy and childbearing occur? (2) How could programs target the teenagers who are at highest risk for premarital pregnancy, for example, nonwhite females in low-income families? (3) How could more basic policy initiatives addressed to the underlying social structural factors that encourage out-of-wedlock childbearing, particularly among young black couples, facilitate pregnancy prevention and intervention programs?

These three questions are crucial for policymakers to consider if they are to avoid repeating mistakes caused by ignorance of or indifference to these issues.

Background Issues

Previous analyses of the complex sociocultural issues involved in black teenage pregnancy have emphasized the concepts of a "culture of poverty" and a "deviant subculture" operating in black low-income inner-city communities and characterized by high rates of delinquency and criminality, drug addiction, long-term welfare dependency, and female-headed families (Clark 1967; Schulz 1969; Glasgow 1981). Some researchers have attempted to demonstrate that these deviant behaviors are replicated over time through the intergenerational transmission of values or behaviors or both, resulting in the development of an urban "underclass" (Hogan and Kitagawa 1985; McLanahan and Bumpass 1986; Ricketts and Sawhill 1986; Vinovskis 1988*b*). However, other researchers have challenged these findings on the grounds that the behaviors represent a realistic response to the continuing social and economic inequities that poor black families have experienced over several generations (Valentine 1968; Wilson 1987). Thus, problems of black teenage pregnancy and welfare dependency cannot be explained solely in terms of a deviant subculture unique to blacks. As documented by studies of other persistently poor groups, poverty itself is associated with a set of symptomatic responses that share similar characteristics across cultures (Lewis 1966*b;* Grønbjerg et al. 1978).

The major weakness of the "culture of poverty" and related concepts is that they fail to distinguish between behaviors that evolve gradually out of a group's adaptation to a particular social and ecological niche (e.g., Appalachian whites) and those behaviors that represent a defensive response to enforced segregation and restricted socioeconomic opportunities (e.g., blacks and Hispanics). For example, the description of the so-called cultural characteristics of poor blacks by Grønbjerg and her colleagues (1978) falls between stereotype and caricature and appears to be based on a very superficial view of a subgroup of blacks in Northern urban ghettos. This theory has limited heuristic value as an explanation of sexual or social behavior among inner-city blacks, since some of the same phenomena are occurring with increasing frequency among middle-class white adolescents (e.g., teenage pregnancy, drug use, delinquency, date rape, etc.). Moreover, as Furstenberg and his colleagues (1987) point out, stereotypes about black teenage mothers as a monolithic group often prevent a more differentiated view of the diversity in their sexual attitudes and behaviors, their competencies and aspirations, their resources and opportunities, their marital and family experiences, and their life-course trajectories.

Notwithstanding the tendency to pathologize and stereotype the behaviors of inner-city blacks, those attitudinal and behavioral differences that can be legitimately identified must be understood in reference to the underlying socioeconomic and structural conditions that foster and reinforce them.

Thus, there is an urgent need to discriminate between so-called deviant or dysfunctional behaviors of individuals and families and the underlying conditions that may foster these behaviors, for example, the economic and social structural conditions. There is also a need to develop a multifactor theory that accounts for the greater vulnerability of certain low-income families and individuals to chronic dysfunction and social deviance, although other families in the same environment manage to function effectively and rear productive children.

The social structural conditions, as outlined by Franklin (1988b), include social welfare policies, national social and economic policies, and employment and unemployment rates for black males and females. Franklin reviews several studies that have demonstrated the relationship between marriage rates of black women and employment rates of black men, showing that female marriage rates have decreased as male unemployment rates have increased. Wilson and Neckerman (1984) have offered the most comprehensive analysis of this relationship, illustrating the attrition of eligible black males through unemployment, incarceration, and self-destructive behaviors. These researchers have coined the term "Male Marriageable Pool Index" (MMPI) to describe the ratio of eligible, employed males to single females at various age levels. It is clear that, at the prime age of family formation (twenty to twenty-four) for black females, they have less than a one in two chance of finding a suitable mate among young black males of the same age-group.

Vinovskis (1988b) criticized Wilson's findings on both conceptual and methodological grounds. Vinovskis points out a number of weaknesses in Wilson's hypothesis that male unemployment rates are correlated to out-of-wedlock birthrates among black adolescents as well as to the proportion of female-headed households in four regions of the country. Vinovskis offers some valid criticisms of Wilson's methodological approach, but his own counterarguments reveal an overly simplistic analysis of the problem. For example, he reports the results of a study showing that, among the eighteen- to twenty-two-year-old black absent fathers, half were employed or in military service. Thus, he asserts that joblessness alone could not account for the fact that 89.7 percent of fifteen- to nineteen-year-old black adolescent births were out of wedlock. What he fails to point out is that most of these young black males work in the "secondary sector" of the economy where wages are low, job benefits are few, and job security is very tenuous (Larson 1988). For those men, the minimum wage is not sufficient to support a wife and child; thus they are not in a much more favorable position to assume responsibility for a family than young men who are in school or unemployed. In fact, young black male high school drop-outs experienced a severe decline of 61 percent in real annual earnings between 1973 and 1984, while their peers who graduated from high school did not fare much better, with a 52 percent drop in real earnings (Children's Defense Fund 1987b). This translates into incomes too low for these young men to support three-person families above the poverty line: only 12 percent of the school drop-outs and 30 percent of the high school graduates with incomes could do so. Further, Vinovskis fails to evaluate the total social context of these young black males and females that could contribute to their reluctance to form families.

In the following section we shall examine this broader social context by documenting the status of young black males in relation to their ability and availability to assume responsibility for a wife and child.

Problematic Status of Young Black Males

Six social indicators have been selected to illustrate the deteriorating status of young black males aged fifteen to twenty-four labeled an "endangered species" in American society (Gibbs 1988*b*). The social indicators are school drop-out rates, unemployment rates, delinquency and crime, substance abuse, homicide, and suicide. This age-group includes young adult males, twenty to twenty-four, who are likely to be the sexual partners of females in their late teens because of an average two-year differential in the ages of young couples in dating relationships. Studies have also found that a high proportion of the fathers of children born to adolescent mothers are in their early twenties (Marsiglio 1987; Robinson 1988).

Although high school completion rates of black youth have improved nationally in recent years, drop-out rates for inner-city black males remain high, approaching levels of 40 to 50 percent (Jaynes and Williams 1989). According to an Urban League study, black males leave school primarily because of family economic problems, academic difficulties, or disciplinary problems (Williams 1982). Inner-city schools have been particularly ineffective in educating black males, whose failures at least partly reflect the widespread problems of poorly prepared teachers, inadequate educational facilities, low teacher expectations, ineffective administrators, and chronic violence (Reed 1988). In 1980, one of five black male teenagers was unable to read at the fourth-grade level and was thus unqualified for most entry-level jobs, apprenticeship programs, or military service. Without a high school diploma or at least basic literacy, these youths are incapable of working at a fast-food restaurant, driving a bus, or stocking shelves at a supermarket.

Then, too, unemployment rates for these inner-city youths range from forty to sixty percent, three times higher than in 1960. Employment rates for black males sixteen to nineteen dropped from 42 percent in 1960 to 36 percent in 1980. In 1984 nearly half of all black youths sixteen to twenty-four had never held a regular job. Black youths bear the brunt of all youth unemployment and still are likely to be "last hired and first fired." When they do work, their jobs are concentrated in the service, manufacturing, and wholesale and retail industries, where they usually occupy positions that require minimal training, have few benefits, and are subject to high turnover rates (Freeman and Holzer 1986; Larson 1988). Such jobs certainly do not offer the kind of job security or mobility that would enhance a young man's prospects for marriage.

Third, crime and delinquency are rampant in the inner cities, with black youths accounting for close to one-third of juvenile arrests for felony offenses, although they represent only one-fifth of the young population. Black youths are also significantly more likely than any other ethnic group to be incarcerated in public juvenile facilities for overall delinquency as well as for violent felony offenses (Krisberg et al. 1986). Thus, they are disproportionately involved in the juvenile justice system at all levels. This entanglement results in severe limitations on their educational and occupational opportunities and creates a vicious cycle of delinquency, incarceration, and recidivism, with the ultimate prospect of a chronic criminal career or marginal social adaptation in adulthood (Krisberg et al. 1986; Dembo 1988). One study predicts that up to 15 percent of all black males will spend some time in an adult prison during their lifetimes, compared to up to 3 percent of white males (Krisberg et al. 1986). Black males with this antisocial background are less likely to form stable family attachments and to be able to fulfill financial obligations for any children, so women who are involved in sexual relationships with them would behave rationally by not marrying them if given that option.

Also, drug abuse is endemic in many inner-city neighborhoods transformed into battlegrounds over the sale and distribution of cocaine and heroin. Data from the National Institute on Drug Abuse (1979) indicates that nonwhite youths (90 percent of whom are black) in the eighteen to twenty-five age-group have higher or equal rates of drug abuse than white youths in every major drug category except inhalants and hallucinogens. The drug industry has not only created lucrative jobs for unemployed teenagers, it has also created a violent life-style and a new health menace for black males. Heterosexual intravenous drug users account for more than one-third of the AIDS cases among black males, who now represent one-fourth of all male cases. Recently there has been a dramatic increase in the number of black females who are infected wih the HIV virus; as of December 1988, 54 percent of all women with AIDS were black heterosexuals, most of whom had contracted it through sharing unsterilized needles or through sexual intercourse with AIDS-infected male drug addicts (Centers for Disease Control 1989).

Epidemiologists have predicted that the incidence of AIDS will continue to increase among young inner-city blacks, who are particularly at risk because of their high rates of drug use and their tendency to engage in unprotected sexual intercourse. Programs of AIDS education and prevention have been slow to penetrate inner-city communities, and some survey and clinical data suggest that low-income black youths have not substantially modified their sexual and social behaviors in response to the threat of this disease (Gibbs 1988b). Moreover, interviews with the pregnant partners of black male AIDS patients indicate an unwillingness to terminate their pregnancies even though there is a 50 percent chance of giving birth to a baby infected with the AIDS virus (Gross 1988). Yet these same women did not expect financial support from their partners and, in most cases, were not married to them. The implication is that, although these women may engage in high-risk patterns of drug use and sexual behaviors, they are still able to make rational judgments about the limited prospects for financial support and marriage from their addicted partners.

In addition, homicide is the leading cause of death among young black males. A young black male has a one in twenty-one chance of being murdered before he reaches age twenty-one, usually by another black male who fires a gun (U.S. Department of Health and Human Services 1986). Young black males are six times as likely as young white males to be victims of homicide. Despite the fact that there has been a decline in the homicide rate for this group since it peaked in 1970 at 102.5 per 100,000, the current rate of 61.5 per 100,000 is still 33 percent higher than it was in 1960. This level of violence indicates a disregard for human life and a profound alienation from shared community norms and values. Further, this high homicide rate creates a climate of violence and fear in inner-city areas where gunfire may erupt at any time over gang fights, drug trafficking, or perceived insults to one's masculinity. Young women who live in these areas must confront the perpetual sense of danger and impermanence, coping with the constant threat of injury or death for themselves or their families (Anderson 1989). Under these conditions, they may view relationships as grounded in the present, with no guarantees for the future; thus no permanent commitment is sought or expected (Schulz 1969; Ladner 1971). These young women have learned through years of painful experience that they must rely upon themselves and that their male partners are vulnerable to unemployment, involvement with the criminal justice system, drug addiction, and unpredictable violence.

Suicide, the final social disorder, is the third leading cause of death for young black males. Since 1960, suicide rates have nearly tripled for this group; while suicide among whites increases with age, it is a peculiarly youthful phenomenon among blacks (Gibbs 1988*a*). Historically, low suicide rates in the black community have been attributed to the cohesiveness of the black family, the influence of the black church, and the importance of social support networks in the black community (Billingsley 1968; Stack 1974; Allen 1978). With all of these institutions weakened through urbanization, poverty, and structural changes in the family, young blacks have had very few, if any, protective buffers to shield them from the many stresses of prejudice and discrimination in this society. In the fifteen to twenty-four age-group, the suicide rate for black males is four times higher than that for black females. This male-female disparity in suicide rates results in a further shortage of available males, particularly in the twenty to twenty-four age-group, where the male-female suicide ratio is even higher than in the fifteen to nineteen age-group.

The cumulative effect of these social indicators, which in each case are more negative for young black males than for black females, has been to reduce the pool of available, employable, and responsible marital partners for black females in the prime years for family formation. However, these social indicators can be viewed more profitably as symptoms of social structural factors in the broader society that contribute to and are reinforced by a set of distinctive sociocultural factors within the black community. These, in turn, get played out through family processes in socialization practices, communication patterns, parental role modeling, and parental control and monitoring of dating behavior (Franklin 1988*b;* Dash 1989). At the individual level, adolescent sexual attitudes and behaviors reflect parental and peer attitudes and are related to the adolescent's general behavioral profile, age of initiating sexual behavior, substance use, school performance, and educational-career aspirations (Jessor and Jessor 1977; Furstenberg et al. 1981; Chilman 1983; Gibbs 1986).

Social Structural Factors

The major social structural factors that have affected black youth and their propensity to form families are the following: (1) structural and technological changes in the economy; (2) government social welfare policies; (3) pervasive discrimination in education, employment, and housing; (4) neighborhood disintegration; (5) differential treatment of black males and females in many sectors of society; and (6) a conservative political climate. Since most of these factors have previously been identified and discussed in depth, they will be briefly summarized, with the emphasis on their relationship to sociocultural factors in the black community.

Structural and technological changes in society have shifted the economy from an agricultural and manufacturing base to a service and high-technology base, requiring a more skilled and educated labor force (Larson 1988). As new jobs have moved from city to suburbs and from East to West, urban black youths have had neither the skills nor the mobility to qualify. For example, the proportion of young blacks who worked year-round fell from 48 percent in 1973 to 32 percent in 1984 (Children's Defense Fund 1987b). Without employment opportunities, they have developed an underground economy in drugs, stolen goods, and gambling.

In addition, scholars have debated the role of government social welfare policies in fostering female-headed families, but most of the studies indicate modest if any effects of welfare policies on adolescent childbearing itself (Ellwood and Bane 1984). In her recent state-by-state analysis of adolescent pregnancy, Singh (1986) found that welfare payments to teenage mothers were negatively associated with birthrates for both black and white adolescent females. However, AFDC payments are associated with greater instability of low-income, two-parent families since current welfare policies do not provide incentives for unemployed fathers to remain in the household (Hoffman and Holmes 1976). This has been a particularly damaging policy for black male household heads, who may be frequently unemployed and perceived as parasites of the system rather than as victims of a changing economy.

Despite the passage of landmark civil rights legislation in 1964 and 1965, a series of Supreme Court decisions striking down discriminatory laws, and presidential executive orders on affirmative action in employment and education, discrimination is still pervasive and persistent in education, employment, and housing. Racial discrimination has been documented in all of these areas, most recently by a study showing that blacks are the most segregated of all groups in their housing patterns, particularly in access to suburban housing (Jaynes and Williams 1989). Over several generations, these patterns of discrimination have resulted in the growth of large urban ghettos, the concentration of blacks in a few lower-paying industries and lower-status occupations, and the development of a de facto system of segregated inner-city schools that have failed to provide adequate education for the majority of black youth (Kasarda 1985; Schorr 1986).

Furthermore, inner-city black neighborhoods have experienced major social upheavals since the early 1960s, when upwardly mobile blacks began moving out of the central city areas into the suburbs (Wilson 1987). This movement, which accelerated with the passage of the civil rights legislation and the increased economic opportunities for educated blacks, had the unintended effect of removing many of the more successful blacks who had provided leadership to the community. As many of these better educated blacks moved out of the inner cities, the communities lost not only their leadership skills but also their stabilizing effects as role models and liaisons to the majority community. The net effort of this social change was that black youth had fewer models of effectively functioning intact families and of successful black adults, and few opportunities to observe diversity in family life-styles and adult occupational roles. In addition, these neighborhoods have experienced high rates of residential mobility, high crime rates, and high levels of stress, all of which are associated with high rates of teen pregnancy (Singh 1986).

Then, too, black males and females have received differential treatment from many institutions and sectors in the dominant society. Compared to black males, black females have generally received more support and encouragement to achieve at all levels of the educational system, they have traditionally been able to find a wider range of employment, and they have had greater access to health and social services (Gibbs 1988a). Society's response to teenage pregnancy offers a good example of the extensive programs and services available to pregnant females as compared to the few available for their male partners (Sander and Rosen 1987; Robinson 1988). This differential treatment is reinforced by socialization strategies of low-income black mothers, who frequently give mixed messages to male children about their marginal status in society and their superfluous role in the family, simultaneously grooming female children to become economically self-sufficient and to assume responsible family roles (Schulz 1969; Ladner 1971).

Finally, an increasingly conservative political climate has fostered a backlash to civil rights advances and affirmative action programs in employment and education. The national debate has shifted from a proactive emphasis on policies of prevention and early intervention to a reactive emphasis on policies of retrenchment and rehabilitation. Unfortunately, young black males have been the major victims of this backlash, as manifested by their higher drop-out rates, their declining college enrollment rates, their increasing unemployment rates, and their falling incomes relative to those of black females (Sum et al. 1987; Larson 1988; Reed 1988) and relative to their socioeconomic status in 1970.

These social structural factors have either contributed to the development of or exacerbated preexisting sociocultural conditions in the black community that in turn, have facilitated the high rates of out-of-wedlock adolescent pregnancy. These factors are discussed in the following section.

Sociocultural Factors

The sociocultural factors identified by Franklin (1988b) and many other scholars as contributing significantly to out-of-wedlock adolescent pregnancy among blacks are poverty; female-headed families; social isolation; neighborhood disequilibrium; cultural attitudes toward sexuality, contraception, and childbearing; and peer cultural values and behaviors. Again, these topics have been amply covered in the social science literature and are reviewed only briefly here.

Nearly one-third of all black families live below the poverty line (U.S. Bureau of the Census 1987a). Nearly half of all black children under eighteen years of age live in poor families. Thus they grow up in substandard housing, attend inferior schools, live in deteriorating neighborhoods, lack access to health care, and are highly exposed to social problems.

For blacks poverty has also meant a special kind of social isolation. They have been forced to live in ghetto communities, to attend segregated schools, and to maintain a separate set of social institutions. This social isolation has inevitably reinforced a set of distinctive values, beliefs, and behaviors adaptive to their environment but sometimes at variance with the values, beliefs, and behaviors of the dominant society (Schulz 1969; Clark 1967; Frazier 1966).

Moreover, this social isolation has enabled blacks to adjust to the changing economic structure by tacitly accepting, if not condoning, the increased number of female-headed families, viewed not as a "deviant" family form but a "variant" family form (Allen 1978; Hogan and Kitagawa 1985). Further, it has fostered the development of folk beliefs about sexuality, contraception, pregnancy, and childbearing that may well have had their roots in the period of slavery, when procreation was one of the major functions of the female slave and children were highly prized not only for their economic value but also for their symbolic survival value for the group (Frazier 1966; Ladner 1971; Thompson 1980; Franklin 1988a; Dash 1989).

Black female-headed families increased from 22 percent in 1960 to 42 percent in 1986 (U.S. Bureau of the Census 1987*b*). Two of every three children (67%) in black female-headed households are poor and welfare dependent. As Wilson and Neckerman (1984) have pointed out, this growth rate parallels the increase in unemployment among black males, which appears to be a major cause of lowered marriage rates in this group. The fact that the current generation of black youth witnessed not only an increase in the number of female-headed families but also an increased community tolerance for that family structure indicates the powerful effect that modeling had on their own conceptions of family structure and parenting roles (McLanahan and Bumpass 1986). In their study of a random sample of over 1,000 black females, aged 13–19, in Chicago, Hogan and Kitagawa (1985) found that "black teenagers from high-risk environments (lower class, resident in a ghetto neighborhood, non-intact family, five or more siblings, a sister who became a teenage mother, and lax parental control of dating) have rates of pregnancy that are 8.3 times higher than girls from low-risk environments" (852).

More specifically, if children grow up in homes where the mother is the self-sufficient household head and there is no stable father figure, girls may receive the implicit message that husbands are not essential to establish and raise a family, and boys may receive the message that one can father children without committing oneself to marriage and child-rearing.

These messages are further reinforced by the sexual attitudes, values, and behaviors of peers and siblings. Several studies have found that teenagers obtain most of their sexual information or misinformation from their peers (Chilman 1983). When that information is delivered in the context of social isolation and absence of sex education programs, it is likely to be inaccurate and to reflect traditional community belief systems. Further, studies have found that girls whose older siblings have had babies are more likely to get pregnant than girls without such a family history (Hogan and Kitagawa 1985; Franklin 1988*b*). Taken together, the influence of peers and siblings has a significant effect on the sexual behaviors and outcomes of black adolescent females—in the direct effects of modeled behaviors and the indirect effects of attitudes, values, and beliefs.

There are two sets of attitudes that require attention for understanding the sexual behaviors of black youth. First, studies of attitudes toward fertility and childbearing indicate that black females express very positive attitudes toward having children and toward pregnancy itself, for example, they express little fear of pregnancy or ambivalence about children (Ladner 1971; Thompson 1980). In my own study of a racially mixed sample of 387 junior high school females, the black subjects expressed more positive attitudes than the whites toward having children in the future. They also expressed expectations of combining marriage and a career with children, and less ambivalence toward this combination than any other group (Gibbs 1986). However, girls with lower educational and career aspirations were significantly more likely to be sexually active younger than girls who had higher aspirations, a finding replicated in many other studies (Moore and Werthheimer 1984; Children's Defense Fund 1988).

The attitudes of black youths toward contraception are less clear-cut. Ethnographic studies indicate that low-income black youths have negative attitudes toward any form of artificial contraception (Schulz 1969; Ladner 1971). However, some surveys have found that, when socioeconomic class is controlled, blacks are as likely as whites to use contraceptives (Robinson 1988). Other studies suggest that black females are as effective as or more effective than whites in using contraception if they are properly instructed (Franklin 1988b). In any case, surveys of adolescent contraceptive practices as well as teenage pregnancy statistics clearly indicate that a large number of black adolescents are not regular and consistent users of contraceptive devices either through lack of knowledge or by conscious choice. This failure to use contraceptives may reflect a number of widely shared folk beliefs that any artificial devices or even birth control pills will cause sterility in women or damage, such as spontaneous abortion or birth defects, to a fetus (Gibbs 1986). Finally, in a study of 13,061 female high school sophomores, 41 percent of whom were black, willingness to consider parenthood was related to patterns of nonconforming behavior and the costs in educational opportunity of becoming a single mother for black females (Abrahamse et al. 1988). Other studies have found that the concept of female "opportunity cost" is an important predictor of fertility rates, for example, "fertility is lowest among women who have the best alternatives to motherhood, and thus perceive the greatest opportunity costs associated with childbearing" (Moore and Werthheimer 1984).

To summarize: a set of sociocultural factors operating in the black family and community have interacted with a set of social structural factors operating in the broader society to facilitate the growth of female-headed families and, in turn, to reinforce the phenomenon of out-of-wedlock teenage pregnancy. Since these sociocultural factors get played out through dynamic family processes, sometimes over several generations, social policies to modify teenage pregnancy and to encourage family formation among black youth can be addressed more effectively to social structural and family levels of intervention.

In the remaining section of this chapter, I shall briefly outline some proposals for social policy initiatives to address both the social structural and the family levels of intervention in order to reduce the incidence of out-of-wedlock teenage pregnancy among blacks and simultaneously to increase the likelihood of family formation among young black couples.

Implications for Social Policy

Much greater attention must be paid to the social context in which adolescent pregnancy, childbearing, and parenting occur in the black community. This context obviously includes the relationship with the child's father, the response of the family, the social attitudes of the community, and the social policies of the society—all will influence the outcomes for the developing child. Social policies should be formulated to take into account all of these factors, but the focus for this chapter is on those policies which will have influence on social structural factors that, in turn, influence sociocultural factors.

First, the federal government needs to develop a full-employment policy to produce sufficient jobs and income for those young adults and teenagers who are in the labor market (Schorr 1986; Larson 1988). Such an employment policy should be coordinated with economic policies that encourage investment in central city areas to stimulate economic growth and to provide new job opportunities for black youths and adults. In this connection, the minimum wage should be raised to a level at which full-time, full-year employment will produce sufficient income to support a family of three above the federal poverty level.

Second, more funds should be allocated for job-training programs and transportation subsidies for those hard-core unemployed young black males who need remedial education, counseling, and job referral information to join the work force. Such programs as the School-to-Work Transition Program, the Job Training Partnership Act (JTPA), and the Job Corps have increased the rates of employment of young black males and have improved their attachment to the labor force (Congressional Budget Office 1982). A stable job and a regular income are prerequisites of supporting a family, so this is probably the single most effective way to increase the supply of marriageable black males.

Third, a comprehensive family assistance policy must be developed for the multiple problems of poor families, many of which are female headed. Such a policy would provide a basic family living standard through direct subsidies or a refundable tax credit, extend coverage to unemployed two-parent families, provide subsidies for low-income housing, provide health coverage and improve access to quality health care, improve adult employment opportunities through work-training programs, and improve educational opportunities for minority children and youth (American Public Welfare Association 1986; Schorr 1986; Edelman 1987). Such policies would virtually eliminate poverty in this country and would enable black families to join the mainstream, to participate in the broader society, and to provide adequate resources for their children. This could be expected to result in better health, higher educational achievement, and lower rates of delinquency, substance abuse, and self-destructive behaviors among black youth.

Fourth, continued legislative and judicial efforts are necessary to eliminate all vestiges of racial discrimination in education, employment, and housing. Aside from the moral, ethical, and legal issues involved in discrimination, it has the invidious effect of creating unequal facilities that become socially isolated from those of mainstream society, thereby creating a climate for the development of intractable social problems, thwarted ambitions, and feelings of alienation, hostility, and despair.

Fifth, the educational system must be restructured to prepare black youth for productive roles in this society. The educational system serving inner-city communities has many severe deficiencies, but four priority areas need to be addressed immediately: (1) the financing of education; (2) curriculum equality; (3) teacher recruitment, training, and placement; and (4) drop-out prevention programs (see Committee for Economic Development 1987). Without education, young black males will not be able to compete in an increasingly technological labor market and they will become expendable. The economy in the twenty-first century will need their productivity, so educating them is a necessity.

Sixth, urban neighborhoods must be redesigned so that housing is integrated both racially and socioeconomically. Then low-income black families could live in areas where there are diverse family life-styles, values, and behaviors. Unfortunately, there is a great deal of resistance to mixed-income, scattered site integrated housing developments, as has been demonstrated in the bitter and long-standing controversies in several localities. However, there are also successful examples of such housing in several metropolitan areas around the country.

If changes are made in these crucial social structural factors, there should be concomitant changes over time in the sociocultural factors implicated in the adolescent pregnancy–childbearing behavioral pattern.

Further, expanded educational and employment opportunities for black youths will help them develop knowledge and skills to play productive roles in society. In addition, conditions will be more conducive for both males and females to develop a sense of competence, a feeling of control over their environment, and a set of career aspirations that will encourage them to delay sexual activity and, consequently, to postpone pregnancy until they are physically, psychologically, and economically prepared to be responsible parents.

In recent years, public policy specialists and politicians have engaged in contentious debate not only about the programs needed to address these problems but also about how they would be financed (Rodgers 1986; Schorr 1986; Danziger and Weinberg 1986; Edelman 1987; Wilson 1989). There is a clear need to articulate a national agenda that places a top priority on eliminating poverty and racism in American society. Legislative initiatives must be funded by reducing expenditures for national defense, reducing the national debt, streamlining foreign aid programs, and closing tax loopholes that favor wealthy individuals and businesses, among other strategies. Model alternative budgets to increase spending on social welfare programs, education, health care, and low-income housing have been proposed by such groups as the Children's Defense Fund (1989) and the Congressional Black Caucus (Parker 1989). Since 1945 the American government has always promptly and magnanimously worked to finance the rebuilding of Asian and European countries after three international wars, to finance the resettlement of political refugees from totalitarian regimes, and to finance the democratization of Eastern European and Third World nations. It is not unreasonable to expect the United States to allocate adequate funds to finance the rebuilding of urban America by supporting programs of prevention and early intervention rather than programs of punishment and rehabilitation, which are costly and less effective in the long run (Schorr 1986; Committee for Economic Development 1987; Edelman 1987).

In conclusion: Anthropologists have emphasized the persistence of values, norms, and behaviors in a given culture. These aspects of culture are very resistant to change and usually change very slowly over a period of several generations. Yet the lesson of rapid social change in developing countries is that there is an interaction between social change and technological change, where certain factors in the social environment create conditions that are favorable to technological change, which, in turn, accelerates the process of social change. When social change occurs in response to technological change, the values, norms, and behaviors of a culture are inevitably affected and evolve over time to adapt to the economic and social changes. If one views the inner-city ghetto as a developing area of society, then one would not expect values and norms to change radically in the absence of any major environmental changes. Thus, to achieve changes in black adolescent sexual attitudes and behaviors, especially in relation to their decisions about pregnancy, childbearing, and parenting, it will be necessary to modify substantially their social and economic environments, to provide them with educational incentives, to enhance their career opportunities, and to increase their access and exposure to the mainstream values and life-styles of American society.

MARK F. TESTA

6 Racial and Ethnic Variation in the Early Life Course of Adolescent Welfare Mothers

Research has long shown that adolescents who assume the maternal role before completing the culturally prescribed transitions of graduating from high school, marrying, or being employed full-time are more likely to be poor and to remain dependent on welfare longer than women who postpone their childbearing. Current estimates are that nearly 60 percent of the women who received Aid to Families with Dependent Children (AFDC) in 1988 were nineteen years old or younger at the birth of their first child (Moore 1990). Recent studies indicate that a good deal of what is defined as "long-term welfare dependency," lasting three consecutive years or more, is concentrated among young, never married mothers (Ellwood 1986; Duncan and Hoffman 1988; Congressional Budget Office 1990). Considering such findings, policymakers have come to see adolescent welfare recipients as a top priority for action to reduce social welfare spending in the United States (Besharov 1989).

The federal Family Support Act of 1988 mandates several policies and programs that are aimed at reducing the welfare dependency of adolescent mothers. Some of these initiatives are benign, such as extending child care assistance for school-age parents; others are quite restrictive, such as requiring labor force participation of mothers with children older than three years and mandating that minor parents live at home as a condition of their eligibility for financial assistance. While one would certainly hesitate to advocate for the right of a minor parent to establish her own household, it is important to acknowledge the paucity of research on the education, work, and family situations of adolescent welfare mothers upon which to base recent policies and programs.

Most previous studies of adolescent welfare dependency have relied on hospital or agency samples composed largely of black adolescent mothers (Klerman and Jekel 1973; Furstenberg and Crawford 1978; Miller 1983). More recent studies using nationally representative samples have been limited to drawing racial comparisons with only a small number of statistical controls, such as age, education, and marital status (Hopkins 1987). Accordingly, it is unknown whether the patterns of welfare usage, school completion, residential mobility, subsequent childbearing, marriage, and employment that have been observed for black adolescent mothers in clinical samples also extend to adolescent mothers of non-Hispanic white, Mexican, and Puerto Rican origins. What is lacking in the literature is "external validation" of past findings with more racially and ethnically diverse samples. The need for greater knowledge about nonblack adolescent welfare mothers is particularly important since demographic and social trends indicate that the problem of adolescent welfare dependency will increasingly become a white and Hispanic phenomenon in the future.[1]

This chapter reports results of the Adolescent Family Life Survey (AFLS) conducted in the early 1980s with a panel of AFDC recipients under eighteen years old in Chicago and suburban Cook County, Illinois. This probability sample of 442 adolescent welfare recipients included an oversampling of non-Hispanic white, Mexican, and Puerto Rican adolescents to permit comparisons with blacks. Recent research finds substantial racial variation in the length of time mothers and children remain dependent on welfare for support (Duncan and Hoffman 1988; Congressional Budget Office 1990). This study reaffirms this finding and extends it to include ethnic variation among Hispanics and whites. All three waves of the panel study showed that black and Puerto Rican adolescent mothers remained dependent on AFDC substantially longer than non-Hispanic white and Mexican mothers. Whereas over one-half (54%) of non-Hispanic white respondents and 39 percent of Mexican respondents moved off the AFDC rolls at least once during the three-year study period, only 24 percent of Puerto Rican and 20 percent of black respondents did so.

What accounts for these racial and ethnic disparities in the duration of welfare dependency? Are they an indication of a deviant subculture or syndrome of behavioral dependency that inhibits economic achievement and social mobility, as some have recently argued (Kaus 1986; Lemann 1986; Novak et al. 1987), or are they a manifestation of the continued denial of economic opportunities and social resources to racial and ethnic minorities (Wilson 1987)? Questions similar to these have long fueled the poverty and welfare debates in the United States (Valentine 1968; Fallers 1973). In this chapter, I shall attempt to move the discussion of adolescent welfare dependency beyond the usual arguments by showing that a large fraction of black adolescents make life-course adaptations to early parenthood that are quite different from the adaptations typically made by white and Hispanic adolescents. Although these adaptations function to prolong the welfare usage of black adolescents longer than that of nonblack adolescents, these patterns cannot rightly be interpreted as arising from wholesale rejection of the values of middle-class achievement. Rather, they are better seen as accommodations to situations of disadvantage that, although departing from mainstream norms, are nonetheless oriented toward achieving educational and economic goals, albeit in nonconventional and risky ways. Policymakers will need to reckon with these alternative life-course adaptations among black adolescents if they are to address successfully the problems of teenage parenthood and welfare dependency in the 1990s.

Culture of Poverty, Social Isolation, or Alternative Life Course

Despite considerable evidence to the contrary, the dominant opinion on the sources of adolescent welfare dependency remains the view associated with the concept of a "culture of poverty" (Valentine 1968; Kaus 1986). Deriving chiefly from the anthropological writings of Lewis (1961; 1966b), this concept holds that the prevalence of early childbearing, nonmarital unions, and reliance on welfare among the poor are features of a self-perpetuating culture of poverty that is antithetical to middle-class norms and values. Lewis attributed the formation of this subculture to the defensive need of the lower class to preserve a sense of dignity under conditions of intense capitalist inequality. More recent journalistic accounts associate these same traits with the lingering effects of a Southern "sharecropping culture" on urban blacks (Lemann 1986; Dash 1989). Whatever the origins, the core idea is that these subcultural norms and values are transmitted intergenerationally through the child socialization practices of the poor and function to inhibit economic achievement and social mobility even after objective opportunities for advancement have improved.

Although Lewis is still cited, few social scientists regard his concept of a culture of poverty as a tenable description of lower-class life (Rainwater 1987). Its popularity has more to do with the "ideology of inequality" that is embraced by the wider society to justify the persistence of poverty than it has to do with the actual behaviors, beliefs, and values of the poor (Fallers 1973). According to its critics, the weaknesses of the concept are its overestimation of the causal significance of the intergenerational transmission of culture (Rainwater 1987) and its underestimation of the prevalence of mainstream values among the poor (Valentine 1968).

In *The Truly Disadvantaged*, Wilson attempts to deal with the former criticism by distinguishing Lewis's concept from the related one of "social isolation." According to Wilson, the concept of social isolation posits a weaker intergenerational effect and a greater responsiveness of behavior to variation in situational constraints and opportunities than does a culture of poverty.

Culture of poverty implies that basic values and attitudes of the ghetto subculture have been internalized and thereby influence behavior. Accordingly, efforts to enhance the life chances of groups such as the ghetto underclass require, from this perspective, social policies (e.g., programs of training and education as embodied in mandatory workfare) aimed at directly changing these subcultural traits. Social isolation, on the other hand, not only implies that contact between groups of different class and/or racial backgrounds is either lacking or has become increasingly intermittent but that the nature of this contact enhances the effects of living in a highly concentrated poverty area. These concentration effects include the constraints and opportunities in neighborhoods in which the population is overwhelmingly socially disadvantaged—constraints and opportunities that include the kinds of ecological niches that the residents of these neighborhoods occupy in terms of access to jobs and job networks, availability of marriageable partners, involvement in quality schools, and exposure to conventional role models. [61]

Wilson's concept of social isolation restores to the poverty debate the importance of neighborhood ecology and peer influences in shaping and reinforcing ghetto-specific behavior. It also holds forth greater promise for the efficacy of liberal reforms than does a culture of poverty. Still, the two concepts are limiting. Both tend to emphasize the pathological or deviant aspects of ghetto-specific culture, such as the inability to delay gratification (Lewis 1961), or welfare as way of life (Wilson 1987), without granting sufficient recognition to its adaptive and positive aspects. Neither adequately allows for the possibility that ghetto-specific culture can include creative adaptations to conditions of disadvantage that facilitate socioeconomic achievement, albeit in nonconventional ways.

The idea of an alternative life course (see Hamburg and Dixon this volume) addresses this limitation by recognizing that certain subcultural patterns, while at variance with mainstream norms, nonetheless may be oriented toward commonly accepted ends. Ethnographic and survey research suggest that out-of-wedlock childbearing among black adolescents may not be as uniformly detrimental to their future well-being as is commonly supposed (Geronimus 1987; Furstenberg et al., this volume). Black families rarely respond to adolescent childbearing by encouraging the young couple to marry but rather allow the girl to remain as a subfamily of her parental household. In some cases, this arrangement will involve the grandmother's informally adopting the infant and raising both the adolescent parent and her child as "siblings." More often, it will involve the grandmother's serving as a "mothering mentor" (Farber 1987) to her daughter, whom she expects to assume many of the responsibilities of parenthood but whom she also allows to participate in normal adolescent activities by providing child care. Both responses allow the adolescent mother the time needed to complete school and to forge the social support networks required before joining the work force when her children reach school age.

In the following sections, I shall examine the extent to which the concept of an alternative life course adequately describes the school, household, and marital transitions made by adolescent welfare mothers from fifteen to twenty years old. I shall compare the typical transitions made by black welfare recipients to those made by white and Hispanic welfare recipients and model the effects of these transitions on the rate of exit from welfare. In the course of this analysis, I shall also introduce three statistical indicators to serve as proxies for the three major explanations of long-term welfare dependency delineated above: (1) whether the respondent's mother was an AFDC recipient herself when the respondent applied for her own grant (culture of poverty); (2) whether many of the respondent's neighbors depend regularly on welfare for support (social isolation); and (3) whether the respondent had aspirations to attend college (alternative life course). While such proxy measures will not permit us to draw firm conclusions about the validity of these respective explanations, the patterns of association we observe should provide a useful guide for future inquiry.

The Adolescent Family Life Survey

The AFLS sample was drawn from a population of pregnant and parenting adolescent mothers, seventeen years old and younger, who were grant recipients or beneficiaries of AFDC in Chicago and suburban Cook County, Illinois. Initial interviews for the three-wave panel study were conducted in 1981 by the Illinois Department of Public Aid, and two follow-up interviews were conducted by NORC, the National Opinion Research Center, in 1983 and 1984. At the two follow-ups, respondents filled out detailed life history calendars recording month-to-month changes in pregnancies and births, education, places of residence, employment, and welfare receipt. The period of observation covered respondents' early life-course development from ages fifteen to twenty years. Just under 70 percent of the original sample participated in all three waves of the survey—a high proportion considering the transience of the adolescent welfare population.

Because of the sample restrictions on age, AFLS respondents were quite young at the time of their first pregnancy. Nearly three-quarters of the sample became pregnant before their sixteenth birthday. While a sample of school-age parents represents a narrow slice of the entire population of teenage parents (less than one-third of teenage births are to minors), there is less selectivity bias by marital status in a sample of parents drawn from welfare rolls at these younger ages than at older ones. Eligibility to receive AFDC in Illinois is limited to unmarried mothers or to married couples with an unemployed wage earner. For this reason, a larger fraction of school-age parents are represented in a welfare sample than older adolescent parents who are more likely to be married.[2]

As expected, most respondents were unmarried at the time of their child's birth (94%) and became beneficiaries of their own AFDC grant at that time or shortly thereafter. The median age of recipience was sixteen and a half years. There was little difference in this statistic by race and ethnicity. A small proportion of respondents chose to remain as child beneficiaries under their mother's grant. But since payments are larger to a family head, most of the school-age mothers (over 95%) eventually applied for benefits as separate assistance units. A small fraction of mothers (less than 5%) received benefits on behalf of their child only.[3]

Also as expected, the selection of the sample from AFDC rolls resulted in a pool of respondents that was relatively homogeneous in class and family origins. Class and family variation by race and ethnicity were greatly restricted. Approximately 80 percent of both black and Puerto Rican respondents reported that their fathers were absent from the home at the time they first became pregnant, as did 70 percent of both non-Hispanic white and Mexican respondents. Among the fathers who were present, between 40 and 60 percent were out of work. Among the mothers who were present in the home, many were themselves current recipients of AFDC: 80 percent of Puerto Ricans, 70 percent of blacks, 60 percent of Mexicans, and 40 percent of non-Hispanic whites.

In contrast to the class and family similarities in the sample, there were large racial and ethnic differences in the spatial distribution of adolescent welfare mothers throughout the Chicago and suburban Cook County areas. Most of the black respondents lived in inner-city Chicago neighborhoods and in public-housing high rises which fan out on the South Side and West Side of the city. Hispanic respondents were concentrated in two areas corresponding to the locations of the largest Puerto Rican and Mexican communities in the city. Meanwhile, non-Hispanic white respondents were scattered throughout the surrounding suburban communities and on the city's North Side. Because Chicago's North Side and suburban neighborhoods are of higher socioeconomic status than the city's West Side and South Side neighborhoods, very few of the non-Hispanic white respondents could be said to reside in poor neighborhoods. Classification of zip codes by whether respondents lived in nonpoverty or poverty areas (defined as having 20% or more of area residents with family incomes below the official poverty line) revealed that only 30 percent of non-Hispanic whites resided in poor neighborhoods. By comparison, 80 percent of Puerto Ricans, 70 percent of blacks, and almost 60 percent of Mexicans lived in neighborhoods that met the census definition of a poverty area.

Racial Variation in Group Adaptations
to Adolescent Parenthood

The AFLS data on the life history of adolescent welfare mothers from fifteen to twenty years old lend support to the concept of an alternative life course among blacks. Even though the ages at which respondents first became pregnant and later became AFDC recipients differed by only a couple of months, there were large racial differences in the ages at which they left school and left their parental homes. The median age for leaving school for blacks (16.6 years old) was a year later than the median ages for non-Hispanic white, Puerto Rican, and Mexican adolescent mothers, and the median age at leaving home for blacks (19.3) was more than two years later. This slower pace of transition from school and home was associated with higher levels of school graduation. At last follow-up, 23 percent of black respondents held a high school diploma, compared to 6 percent or less of non-Hispanic white, Puerto Rican, and Mexican respondents. Some of the racial differences in educational completion and residential independence were tied to a higher probability of marriage among nonblack respondents. During the study period, 37 percent of non-Hispanic white, 27 percent of Mexican, and 19 percent of Puerto Rican respondents had ever married compared to only 8 percent of black respondents.

Table 6.1 provides descriptive data on the different patterns of adaptation to adolescent childbearing among racial and ethnic groups in the AFLS sample. I classified respondents by whether they were still attending school three months after the birth of their first child and by whether they had left home or married before turning eighteen. This led to my identifying five different types of group adaptations to adolescent parenthood, ranging from what may be termed the alternative life course (stayed in school and in the parental home) to the traditional response (left school and married). Four cases did not fit into any of these five categories and are omitted from the tabulations.

The cross-classification of respondents by race and ethnicity and type of adaptation clearly reveals the large racial differences in life-course adaptations to adolescent parenthood. The modal response of blacks (45%) was the alternative life-course adaptation of staying in school and residing with parents. The modal response of nonblacks was nearer to the traditional dropping out of school, establishing a separate household, and eventually marrying; but only a minority of nonblacks (about 17%) completed the transition to marriage before turning eighteen. Comparing the five different patterns shows that the alternative life-course adaptation was associated, at last interview, with the highest high school or GED completion (47%) and the fewest births (1.6 per woman) but with the lowest rate of AFDC exit (17%) and the next highest rate of continued or renewed dependence on welfare (87%). In contrast, the traditional marital adaptation was associated with next to the lowest high school or GED completion (12%) and the most births (1.9 per woman) but with the highest rate of AFDC exit (58%) and the lowest rate of continued or renewed dependence on welfare (71%).

The sizable degree of racial variation in the early life-course adaptations and transitions of adolescent welfare mothers shows that there are characteristic differences between the paths that black adolescent wel-

TABLE 6.1

Life-Course Adaptations to Adolescent Childbearing by Race, Ethnicity, and Status at Last Interview

	STILL IN SCHOOL 3 MOS. AFTER CHILDBIRTH		LEFT SCHOOL BEFORE OR WITHIN 3 MOS. AFTER CHILDBIRTH		
CHARACTERISTICS	Lived with parents as minor	Lived apart from parents as minor	Lived with parents as minor	Lived apart from parents as minor	Married before 18
Weighted percentage	37.7%	14.0%	27.8%	16.5%	4.0%
Sample N	128.	55.	123.	121.	39.
ROW PERCENTAGES					
Black	44.6%	14.7%	27.5%	11.6%	1.6%
Puerto Rican	3.2%	6.3%	23.8%	50.8%	15.9%
Mexican	6.4%	14.9%	21.3%	40.4%	17.0%
Non-Hispanic white	8.2%	6.1%	27.6%	40.8%	17.3%
MEANS					
Age at last interview	19.8	19.8	20.3	20.0	20.2
Births per woman	1.6	1.9	1.7	1.8	1.9
PERCENTAGES					
Ever exited AFDC	17.3%	25.4%	18.8%	32.8%	58.3%
Still on welfare at last interview	86.5%	83.6%	89.9%	81.8%	71.0%
High school diploma/GED	47.4%	24.2%	13.3%	4.2%	12.4%
Married at last interview	3.9%	3.6%	6.4%	8.9%	30.8%

fare mothers are likely to take to maturity and the paths that white and Hispanic welfare mothers are likely to take. Black respondents are more likely to remain in the parental home, continue in school, and delay marriage, while white and Hispanic respondents are more likely to leave the parental home, drop out of school, and marry. Because continuation in school extends AFDC elibility while early marriage cuts it short, the possibility must be considered that it is primarily this difference in life-course adaptations to early childbearing that explains racial variation in the persistence of adolescent welfare dependency rather than a culture of poverty or social isolation. To shed some light on the relative strengths of these three explanations of prolonged welfare dependency, I turn next to a discussion of findings from a multivariate analysis of the effects of various risk factors on age-specific rates of exit from AFDC.

Racial and Ethnic Variation in Rates of Welfare Exit

Because only a portion of the life span of respondents was recorded during the AFLS period of study, the length of time that adolescent mothers received AFDC was only partly observed. While complete durations of initial welfare spells were known for the 30 percent of respondents who left the AFDC program at least once during the study period, the full durations were unknown for the remaining 70 percent. I therefore used a statistical method that makes allowances for the fact that portions of the welfare histories of respondents are missing, or "censored," to use the statistical terminology. This method, which has become common in life history investigations, is hazards regression analysis.[4]

Table 6.2 summarizes the results of the analysis. The models are statistical estimations of the average relationship between the likelihood of welfare exit and a person's classification on the set of risk factors listed in table 6.2. The specific quantities in this table are estimates of relative risks and can be interpreted as multipliers of a comparison group's age-specific probability of exiting AFDC (which is fixed at 1). A relative risk larger than 1 indicates a greater tendency toward exiting AFDC than the comparison group, while a relative risk smaller than 1 indicates a lesser tendency. A relative risk equal or close to 1 indicates the same tendency as the comparison group. Quantities that are marked with three asterisks are sufficiently different from 1.0 to pass a test of statistical significance at the 0.01 level. Since very few respondents had ever married before receipt of AFDC (6%), married or previously married women are omitted from the analysis.

Model 1 indicates that there are sizable racial and ethnic differences in the age-specific rates at which never-married adolescent mothers leave the AFDC program. The relative risks show that blacks leave welfare at

TABLE 6.2

Relative Risks of First Welfare Exits by Race and Ethnicity

	RELATIVE RISKS				
	All groups			Blacks	Whites and Hispanics
	MODELS				
RISK FACTOR LEVEL	1	2	3	3A	3B
Race/ethnicity					
Black	0.27***	0.40***	0.48***		
Puerto Rican	0.44*	0.71	1.04		0.87
Mexican	0.91	1.26	1.18		0.97
Non-Hispanic white	1.	1.	1.		1.
AFDC grant benefits					
Child only	3.63***	3.60***	5.63***	6.08***	5.50***
Adult and child	1.	1.	1.	1.	1.
Education of mother					
8th grade or less	0.61*	0.50***	0.37***	0.35**	0.47**
Above 8th grade	1.	1.	1.	1.	1.
Mother on welfare					
Yes		0.51***	0.44***	0.34*	0.54**
No		1.	1.	1.	1.
Neighbors on welfare					
Many		0.67*	0.64*	0.82	0.46**
Not many		1.	1.	1.	1.
College aspirations					
Yes		0.54***	0.48***	0.48*	0.52**
No		1.	1.	1.	1.
High school drop-out					
Yes			1.51	1.49	1.69
No, graduated			5.53***	6.03***	4.36*
No, still in school			1.	1.	1.
Independent household formation					
Yes, premarital			1.64**	1.30	1.68
Yes, postmarital			25.21***	24.44***	27.39***
No, still at home			1.	1.	1.
Employment					
Employed			5.45***	5.04***	7.45***
Not employed			1.	1.	1.
N	412	372	372	216	156
Censored	72%	72%	72%	81%	60%

Note: All models include indicators of respondent's age at the start of welfare receipt (relative risks not reported in table).
***$p<0.01$ **$p<0.05$ *$p<0.10$

approximately one-fourth (0.27) the rate of non-Hispanic whites (the baseline comparison group); Puerto Ricans leave at a slightly higher rate (0.44); and Mexicans leave at nearly the same rate as whites (0.91). Over time, these differences in exit rates translate into lengthier spells of welfare dependency for blacks and Puerto Ricans and much shorter spells for non-Hispanic whites and Mexicans.[5]

The racial and ethnic differences under model 1 are partially adjusted for variation in socioeconomic status; the indicators used are the education of the respondent's mother and the type of AFDC benefit received. Both factors are associated with rates of welfare exit. Respondents whose mother attained no more than an eighth grade education tended to leave AFDC at a 39 percent lower rate than respondents whose mother had more education.[6] Similarly, respondents who were eligible for child benefits exited at only over three and a half (3.63) times the rate of mothers who received benefits for both herself and her child. Besides suggesting that adolescents from higher-income homes have an easier time leaving the welfare rolls, this result may also indicate that some adolescent mothers rely on AFDC primarily for short-term cash assistance and health coverage for their infant under Medicaid. To examine the extent to which other factors besides socioeconomic status may help to explain the higher rates of welfare exits among non-Hispanic white and Mexican adolescent welfare recipients compared to black and Puerto Rican recipients, model 2 introduces proxy indicators for the three major explanations of long-term welfare dependency delineated above: (1) culture of poverty, (2) social isolation, and (3) alternative life course. The results are as follows.

Prior welfare receipt by the respondent's family (a proxy for culture of poverty) is associated with lower exit rates. Respondents who reported that their mothers were already recipients of AFDC at the time they applied for their own beneifts tended to leave AFDC at a 49 percent lower rate than respondents whose mothers were not welfare recipients. This is the result that one would predict if welfare dependency was transmitted intergenerationally. Adolescents from welfare-dependent families would remain longer on AFDC than low-income adolescents whose families were not dependent on welfare.

Living in a welfare-dependent neighborhood (a proxy for social isolation) is only weakly associated with lower exit rates. Respondents who reported that many of their neighbors depend regularly on welfare for support tended to exit the welfare rolls at a 33 perent lower rate than adolescents who lived in less impoverished areas. This is the result one would predict if social isolation constrained social mobility. Adolescent mothers from disadvantaged neighborhoods would have fewer opportunities to achieve self-sufficiency through education, employment, or marriage than low-income adolescents from less disadvantaged neighborhoods.

Finally, college aspirations (a proxy for the alternative life course) prolong rather than shorten welfare dependency. Respondents who reported at the first interview that they planned to attend college had a 46 percent lower exit rate than adolescents with lower educational aspirations. This result runs contrary to the stereotypical notion that welfare dependency is related to a lack of motivation. This is the result that would be predicted if AFDC functioned as a sort of an "educational stipend" to enable adolescent parents to continue their education as an alternative to marriage or full-time employment.

Even though each of the explanations of long-term welfare dependency receives provisional support from the analysis thus far, no one factor alone accounts for much of the racial and ethnic variation in welfare exit rates. When they are considered jointly, however, a good deal of the ethnic variation is explained. The relative risks for Mexicans and Puerto Ricans are statistically indistinguishable from non-Hispanic whites'. In comparison, only about 18 percent of the difference in the relative risk associated with race is explained by these factors. The racial difference diminishes further with the introduction of the life-course variables under model 3, but again the change is modest. The inclusion of school, household, marriage, and employment transitions into the analysis raises the amount of explained racial variation to about 29 percent. By comparison, the inclusion of life-course variables wipes out the remaining difference between non-Hispanic whites and Puerto Ricans. Most of the ethnic variation in the persistence of welfare dependency among whites and Hispanics apparently is explainable by these socioeconomic and life-course variables.

The life-course transition most strongly associated with welfare exit rates is marriage, followed by high school graduation and then employment. When they are considered jointly, however, the multiplicative effect of joining the work force with a high school diploma ($5.53 \times 5.45 = 30.14$) exceeds the effect associated with marriage alone. Forming an independent household before marriage does not appear to elevate seriously the risk of an adolescent mother's remaining on welfare relative to her staying in her parental home. In fact, there is a statistically significant, positive effect of premarital household formation on welfare exit rates. As shown below, however, this apparent effect is confined solely to whites and Hispanics and may reflect unmeasured changes in household income caused by the adolescent's establishing a separate residence with a boyfriend or other person.

The inability of model 3 to account more completely for the racial difference in the duration of adolescent welfare dependency suggests that there are other unmeasured variables that are creating the difference that need to be incorporated into the model. Although this would require additional data collection, I did experiment with including the birth of a second child into the analysis, but there were no changes in any of the estimates. Another interpretation for the racial difference is that it reflects dissimilarities in the behavior responses of black and nonblack adolescents to early life-course transitions and socioeconomic situations. In order to examine whether the welfare responses are similar or different for blacks and nonblacks, I estimated model 3 separately for the two subsamples. These results are also included in table 6.2.

The results show that, with the exception of premarital household formation, each of the modeled influences of high school graduation, marriage, and employment on AFDC exit rates is very similar in both racial groups. This seems plausible, given that the rules regulating AFDC eligibility operate uniformly. Also, the relative risks associated with maternal education, family welfare dependency, and college aspirations retain their same numerical importance in the separate analyses by race. For the most part, the welfare responses to early life-course transitions and socioeconomic conditions appear to be the same in both racial groups. The one risk factor, however, that does differ in the separate analyses is the significance of residing in a disadvantaged neighborhood. Unlike the situation for whites and Hispanics, coming from a heavily welfare-dependent neighborhood appears to have little consequence for the welfare mobility rates of blacks. Even eliminating the life-course variables does not alter the significance of the neighborhood effect. This result raises some doubts about the validity of the social isolation explanation of racial differences in welfare mobility rates, at least as it pertains to neighborhoods. To the extent that social opportunities are fewer for black than for nonblack adolescent mothers in Chicago and suburban Cook County, it appears, on the basis of these data, that racial isolation rather than spatial concentration in impoverished neighborhoods is the more crucial source of the disparity.

School Drop-out, Independent Household Formation, and Marriage

The analysis thus far shows that racial variation in welfare exit rates is partly attributable to group differences in transition rates to high school graduation and marriage. Both positively contribute to adolescents' moving from welfare dependency to financial independence. As documented previously, black adolescent welfare mothers are more likely to prolong their dependence on AFDC by following the longer educational route to self-sufficiency, while non-Hispanic white and Mexican adolescent welfare mothers are more likely to cut it short by taking the marital route. The analysis also shows that racial variation in welfare exit rates is partly attributable to group differences in socioeconomic status as measured by maternal education, family welfare history, and college aspirations. To examine the extent to which these risk factors operate similarly on school and marital transitions for both racial groups, I estimated the relative risks of adolescent mothers making these transitions, again using hazards regression to handle the problem of censored observations.

Table 6.3 reports the findings. The data show some important similarities across racial groups. The school drop-out rate is similarly related in both subsamples to the educational status of the adolescent's mother and to her own educational aspirations. Adolescents whose mother had an eighth grade education or less were more likely to leave school prematurely, and adolescents with plans to attend college were less likely to leave. The data also show some important differences. Marriage rates are significantly related to neighborhood only for white and Hispanic adolescents, and school drop-out rates are virtually identical for black adolescents who reside in heavily welfare-dependent neighborhoods compared to those who do not. The absence of a sizable neighborhood effect among blacks agrees with the previous results for welfare mobility rates. Finally, the results on the intergenerational effects of family welfare dependency suggest little relationship. Neither dropping out of school nor marriage is strongly or consistently related to whether the respondent's mother was already an AFDC recipient at the time she first became pregnant.

The absence of a strong association between maternal welfare dependency and the respondent's educational and marital behaviors raises some doubt about the validity of interpreting the effect of this risk factor on welfare exit rates as evidence for a culture of poverty. To be fair, my analysis is limited to the postbirth experiences of a selective population of adolescent welfare mothers, and I cannot be confident that the association is also weak for the entire population of adolescents. Nonetheless, one may have imagined that an intergenerational culture of poverty would act indirectly on welfare mobility rates by increasing school drop-out rates or reducing transitions to marriage. The relative risk of dropping out of school or marriage that was tied to maternal welfare history, however, was insignificant in both subsamples.

TABLE 6.3

Relative Risks of School Drop-out and Marriage by Race and Ethnicity

	RELATIVE RISKS			
	SCHOOL DROP OUT		MARRIAGE	
	Blacks	Whites and Hispanics	Blacks	Whites and Hispanics
RISK FACTOR LEVEL	MODELS 1	2	3	4
Ethnicity				
Puerto Rican		0.68		0.20***
Mexican		0.77		0.67
Non-Hispanic white		1.		1.
Pregnancies and births				
One child	1.	1.	1.	1.
Second pregnancy	1.44	1.10	1.31	0.90
Two children	2.72***	1.17	0.87	1.40
Education of mother				
8th grade or less	1.65**	1.71	0.62	1.0
Above 8th grade	1.	1.	1.	1.
Mother on welfare				
Yes	1.52	0.69	0.48	0.76
No	1.	1.	1.	1.
Neighbors on welfare				
Many	1.22	2.55	1.52	0.52*
Not many	1.	1.	1.	1.
College aspirations				
Yes	0.66*	0.48	1.80	0.76
No	1.	1.	1.	1.
High school drop-out				
Yes			6.59*	4.43
No, graduated				
No, still in school			1.	1.
Independent household formation				
Yes, premarital	2.95***	3.26**	1.86	0.72
Yes, postmarital	1.76	31.10**		
No, still at home	1.	1.	1.	1.
Employment				
Employed	1.22	1.15		0.80
Not Employed	1.	1.		1.
N	224	181	225	182
Censored	25%	6%	92%	71%

Note: All models include indicators of respondent's age at first birth (not reported in table). Empty cells indicate factors not estimated in the model.
***p<0.01 **p<0.05 *p<0.10

I also examined the relationship between maternal welfare dependency and more direct indicators of a culture of poverty, such as the acceptability of welfare, low educational aspirations, and intentional pregnancies, but again I found no association. Whether the significant relationship reported in the previous section between maternal welfare dependency and welfare exit rates is indeed indicative of an adolescent's socialization into a culture of poverty or merely correlated with unmeasured financial disadvantage or sample selection biases will require further evaluation.

One of the strongest relationships in table 6.3 is between dropping out of school and independent household formation. This agrees with the descriptive findings presented in table 6.1. Adolescent welfare mothers who moved away from their paternal home were three times more likely to disrupt their education as adolescents who remained at home. This relationship holds for nonblacks and blacks. In addition, white and Hispanic adolescent mothers who established separate households upon marrying were over thirty times more likely to drop out of school. The low relative risk of dropping out for married black adolescents reflects the small number of black marriages and the fact that school drop-out usually preceded marriage. The marriage model shows that the relative marital risk for black adolescents who dropped out of school was almost seven times as large as the risk for blacks who stayed in school. The effect of dropping out of school on marriage is similar but less pronounced among whites and Hispanics.

These results point to the incompatibility between independent household formation and high school graduation among adolescent welfare mothers. Respondents who moved out of their parental homes on their own or with a husband were much less likely to graduate from high school than those who remained with their parents. This suggests the importance of parental support to the viability of the alternative life course for whites and Hispanics as well as blacks (see Rosenheim, this volume). Separation from the parental home attenuates the sorts of support adolescent welfare mothers can obtain from their parents and adds to the difficulty of balancing child-care needs against classroom demands. For whites and Hispanics, the addition of marital responsibilities imposes extra burdens, while for blacks, the birth of a second child hastens their withdrawing from school. The low drop-out risks for whites and Hispanics who have a second child reflects the fact that, unlike blacks, very few white and Hispanic adolescents managed to remain in school after the birth of their first child (less than 20%).

These results suggest that remaining a student and becoming a wife are competing roles for most adolescent welfare mothers. To what extent is this choice between education or marriage simply a result of differences in the exercise of individual preferences? Although white and Hispanic adolescent welfare mothers tended to leave school and their parental homes at roughly the same ages, they were not all equally likely to marry. Table 6.3 shows that, when other risk factors are statistically controlled, Puerto Rican mothers were only one-fifth (0.20) as likely to marry as non-Hispanic whites. This is approximately the same relative risk that is estimated for blacks when they are compared to non-Hispanic whites in a combined analysis of the two subsamples. Comparison of actual marriage rates to the marriage expectations of respondents at the time they first became pregnant shows a strong interrelationship between these variables. It also shows that, regardless of marriage expectations at pregnancy, non-Hispanic white adolescent mothers were from three to four times more likely to marry than black and Puerto Rican adolescent mothers. Whereas 57 percent of non-Hispanic whites who expected to marry the father of their first child ever married, only 18 percent of black and Puerto Rican adolescents with similar expectations did so. Mexican adolescents were a little less likely to marry (43%) than whites. These are essentially the same results one obtains by entering marriage expectation as an indicator variable in a hazards regression analysis of marital transitions.

The greater ability of non-Hispanic whites and Mexicans to act on their expectations of marriage suggests that black and Puerto Rican adolescent mothers may be facing very different economic and social constraints on their chances for an early marriage. However, the exact nature of these constraints remains elusive. Research on the relationship between male employment status and marriage finds a significant association but one not large enough to explain racial and ethnic differences (Testa et al. 1989; Ellwood 1990). Additional research is needed to assess whether ethnic variation in the acceptance of early marriages plays a significant role. About 19 percent of non-Hispanic white, 17 percent of Mexian, and 16 percent of Puerto Rican adolescent welfare mothers stated that they intentionally became pregnant with the expectation of marrying the father, compared to only 5 percent of blacks. This suggests that for some whites and Hispanics, early pregnancy may be part of a deliberate life-course strategy to accelerate their transition to adulthood by precipitating early marriage and emancipation from parental control. But, as the low marriage figures in table 6.1 indicate, it is a strategy with increasingly uncertain payoffs. Less than 10 percent of the minors who moved out of their parental home were married at the last interview, and only 31 percent of respondents who married as minors were still married.[7]

Public Policy
and Adolescent Welfare Dependency

The Family Support Act of 1988 contains special provisions to deal with the welfare dependence of minor and older adolescents. The Act replaces the existing AFDC program with a program to encourage and assist welfare recipients to obtain the education, training, and employment needed to avoid long-term welfare receipt. One of its implicit goals is to move adolescent welfare recipients along the pathway that I have equated with the alternative life course—continuing in school and remaining in the parental home. The Act seeks to accomplish this goal by (1) requiring as a condition of eligibility that unmarried minor parents live in a place of residence maintained by a parent, legal guardian, or other adult relative; and (2) requiring that custodial parents under twenty years old who have not completed high school participate on a full-time basis in educational activities directed toward the attainment of a high school diploma or its equivalent.

The AFLS data indicate that a substantial proportion of adolescent welfare recipients were already embarked on this path before the passage of the Act. The weighted proportion of adolescents who stayed in school after their child's birth and continued to reside in their parental home as minors was about 38 percent. This pattern, however, was typical only of black adolescent mothers, who constitute about 80 percent of the adolescent welfare caseload in Chicago and suburban Cook County, Illinois. Almost 45 percent of black adolescent recipients stayed in school and lived at home compared to 8 percent of non-Hispanic whites, 6 percent of Mexicans, and only 3 percent of Puerto Ricans. This tight association with race raises the possibility that the viability of the alternative life-course adaptation may depend importantly on a cultural heritage of communal tolerance and extended family support for unmarried mothers and their children among black Americans (see Franklin, this volume). To what extent should or can this adaptation be mandated for whites and Hispanics? As the data showed, only a small percentage of white and Hispanic mothers remained both in school and in their parental home as minors. Most moved out of their parental home shortly after childbirth. The extent to which this racial difference reflects alternate norms about the acceptability of premarital pregnancy, other attitudes about the nature of parental responsibilities after a daughter has children, or differences in the circumstances underlying childbirth to minors will require careful consideration as welfare administrators start enforcing the residence and educational requirements of the Family Support Act.

The other finding—that welfare dependency during adolescence is prolonged by an adolescent's staying in school and remaining in her parental home—suggests that administrators and policymakers need to be cautious about using statistics on short-term welfare terminations when measuring success. The greater the degree to which adolescent welfare mothers adhere to an alternative life course of delaying marriage, living with their parents, and staying in school, the longer they are likely to remain dependent on welfare, at least in the short run, than adolescents who drop out of school, leave home, and marry. Furthermore, the finding that adolescent welfare mothers with college aspirations also tend to remain dependent on AFDC longer than adolescents with lower educational aspirations suggests that modifying ambitions about continuing or returning to school may actually lessen recipients' motivations to leave AFDC until their educational goals have been achieved. Thus, as federal interventions seek to elevate educational aspirations, discourage independent household formation, and increase school continuation rates, the short-term consequences may very well be to increase rather than to decrease the duration of adolescent welfare receipt.

The question of whether an alternative life course is less costly to the public in the long run will not be answerable until more follow-up data from the 1990s can be collected. One sobering fact from the data already in hand is that the promised gains of an alternative life course are not easily achieved. Over a half (53%) of adolescent welfare mothers who were still in school three months after giving birth and who lived at home as minors still lacked a high school diploma at last interview (see table 6.1). Most (87%) continued to draw AFDC checks. Undoubtedly, there will be improvements as the formal services authorized by the Family Support Act are put in place. Still, one potential liability that needs to be considered is whether the semi-institutionalization of an alternative life course among early parents may function inadvertently to bolster current levels of teenage childbearing. If one considers that economic hardship will most likely continue to constrain the marital opportunities of inner-city women, even among those in their mid-twenties, it may seem sensible to some to initiate childbearing earlier rather than later. This way they can draw on the support of government and relatives in raising their children, while simultaneously completing their education and establishing the informal networks needed for full-time labor force participation when their children attain school age. Although it is too soon to assess the plausibility of this argument, the rise in nonmarital childbearing rates among minority adolescents in the late 1980s suggests that policymakers may need to weigh carefully the implications of an alternative life course if they are to address successfully the problems of adolescent parenthood and welfare dependency in the 1990s. This is not meant to imply that the supports should be withdrawn but to caution that serious attention also needs to be paid to redressing those social inequities that make, in the first place, the alternative life course an option conceivably preferable to more conventional pathways to maturity.

Conclusion

Adolescent welfare recipients have become a top priority for action to reduce social welfare spending in the United States. Most of the research on which to base policies and programs, however, has been confined to hospital or agency samples composed largely of black adolescent mothers or to national probability samples with limited data beyond demographic variables for drawing comparisons. Hence, the extent to which the relationships observed for black adolescent mothers in clinical samples also extend to adolescent mothers of white and Hispanic origins is unknown. In this chapter, I have sought to broaden our knowledge of racial and ethnic variation in patterns of adolescent welfare dependency by analyzing survey data from a three-wave panel study of adolescent AFDC recipients in Chicago and suburban Cook County, Illinois.

The data show large racial and ethnic differences in the duration of adolescent welfare dependency, despite the initial similarities in the age, family background, and socioeconomic status of the respondents. At last interview, twice as many non-Hispanic white and Mexican respondents had ever left the AFDC program as Puerto Rican and black respondents. Popular explanations of welfare dependency equate long-term reliance on public aid with a culture of poverty or with social isolation in economically depressed neighborhoods. My analysis shows that these explanations do not satisfactorily describe the conditions associated with the duration of AFDC receipt among adolescent mothers.

I found that welfare recipients who remained in school, lived with their parents, and delayed marriage tended to stay dependent on welfare longer during their adolescence than welfare mothers who dropped out of school, left home, and married. The former pattern, which is consistent with the hypothesis of an alternative life course among blacks, was most typical for black respondents; the latter pattern was most typical for non-Hispanic whites. In order to evaluate more fully the relevance of an alternative life course for understanding racial variation in the duration of adolescent welfare dependency, I modeled the effects of life-course transitions and other factors on the rate of exit from welfare. Three statistical indicators served as proxies for the major explanations of long-term welfare dependency: (1) whether a respondent's mother was already an AFDC recipient at the time of the respondent's first pregnancy (culture of poverty); (2) whether many of the respondent's neighbors depend regularly on welfare for support (social isolation); and (3) whether the respondent had college aspirations (alternative life course).

The analysis showed that controlling for the above risk factors and for the different ages at major life-course transitions explained most of the ethnic differences in welfare exit rates among nonblacks but only a third of the racial difference. Residence in a heavily welfare-dependent neighborhood was associated with lower rates of exit from the AFDC program, but this effect was restricted to white and Hispanic adolescent recipients. Social isolation, as measured by the respondent's perception of neighborhood welfare dependency, did not register as a significant risk factor for long-term welfare dependence among black adolescent mothers. On the other hand, prior welfare receipt by the respondent's mothers was strongly related to reduced rates of welfare exit among both black and nonblack respondents. Although this indication of an intergenerational welfare link appeared to lend support to the concept of a culture of poverty, its lack of association with other life-course transitions, such as school completion and marriage, and with more direct indicators of a culture of poverty, raised doubts about the validity of this concept. The limited relevance of the concept was further reinforced by the finding that adolescent welfare mothers with college aspirations tended to remain longer on AFDC than adolescents with lower educational aspirations. Although this result runs contrary to common stereotypes, it is consistent with my finding that adolescents mothers who adhered to an alternative life course of staying in school, living with their parents, and delaying marriage remained dependent longer on welfare, at least during their adolescence, than adolescents who dropped out of school, left home, and soon married. High school graduation was strongly dependent on adolescent welfare recipients' remaining in their parental homes and delaying marriage.

These results provide a useful counterpoint to the common stereotype of adolescent welfare mothers, especially inner-city black mothers, as mostly alienated from conventional goals of middle-class achievement and hopelessly mired in a culture of poverty or syndrome of behavioral dependency. Although there is little to be gained by denying the reality of these problems for some segment of the adolescent welfare population, it is noteworthy that a sizable percentage of adolescent welfare recipients in Chicago and Cook County, Illinois, were still attending school three months after childbirth and were continuing to reside in their parental homes as minors. Furthermore, almost half of these young women managed to earn a high school diploma or its equivalent by age twenty. What the trade-offs are in expanding and institutionalizing this alternative life course among early mothers may emerge as one of the major policy questions of the 1990s.

NOTES

This research was supported by grants from the Illinois Department of Public Health, the Department of Public Aid, and the Office of Adolescent Pregnancy Programs, U.S. Department of Health and Human Services (APR 000909-02-0). This paper benefited from useful comments by James Coleman and Marta Tienda.

1. This prognosis follows straightforwardly from the fact nonmarital childbearing is already at the saturation point among black adolescent mothers. Virtually all black adolescent mothers are unmarried at the births of their children, and most already rely on public assistance. By comparison, less than half of white and Hispanic adolescent mothers are unmarried at the births of their children. To the extent that the same economic and technological factors that are prolonging the economic dependency of black youth are also affecting other low-income groups, one should expect to see the ratio of nonmarital childbearing continuing to rise among white and Hispanic adolescent parents, and more of these parents turning to welfare for support. If this happens, white and Hispanic adolescent mothers will constitute an ever-increasing fraction of the future adolescent welfare population in the United States.

2. Congressional Budget Office (1990) tabulations of data from the National Longitudinal Survey of Youth (1979–1985) show that 58 percent of mothers under eighteen started receiving AFDC within five years of their first child's birth compared to 43 percent of mothers eighteen to nineteen years old.

3. In Illinois in 1981, the formula for determining whether an adolescent mother was eligible to receive AFDC and Medicaid benefits for her infant depended solely on her financial situation. Her own eligibility for cash assistance depended on her parents' financial situation so long as she was under majority age and remained in her parents' household. A little under 5 percent of AFLS respondents were ineligible for more than child benefits only because of parental income.

4. The key concept of this method is the hazard or transition rate which refers to the conditional probability that an event or transition occurs at a specific time in a person's life. Intuitively, it can be thought of as the risk level for experiencing an event or transition at a given moment. The higher the risk level, the most likely the event or transition is to occur; the lower the risk level, the less likely. Risk levels are assumed to be influenced by a number of factors. Some risk

factors are considered fixed or constant over the period of life examined, such as race and ethnicity. Others, such as births, vary over time. Since many of the time-varying factors that affect movement off welfare, such as school completion, marriage, or employment, are strongly influenced by an adolescent's age, my analysis uses age as the underlying measure of time following a method recommended by Breslow et al. (1983). Because subjects become parents or welfare grantees at different ages in the AFLS sample, membership in the risk set at a given age needs to reflect additions as well as deletions. This method controls for membership by including subjects in the risk set only after they become welfare recipients (for the welfare mobility analysis) or become parents (for other analyses).

5.   My use of age as the underlying measure of time differs from other hazard regression analyses of welfare dependency that use duration of AFDC receipt as the measure of time. Both methods of analysis, however, yield almost identical results when indicators of the respondent's age at welfare receipt are included as fixed covariates in the analyses.

6.   The percentage of change in the exit rate which is associated with a unit change in a risk factor can be calculated by subtracting the relative risk from 1 and multiplying by 100.

7.   This percentage should not be interpreted as indicating that two-thirds of the marriages of minors dissolve. Since unemployment, divorce, or separation is a condition of AFDC eligibility, the AFLS sample excludes most stably employed, married adolescent parents.

FRANK F. FURSTENBERG, JR., MARY ELIZABETH
HUGHES, and JEANNE BROOKS-GUNN

7 The Next Generation: The Children of Teenage Mothers Grow Up

Poverty has been rediscovered in America. It was last rediscovered at the beginning of the Kennedy administration, when the United States was still basking in the afterglow of postwar prosperity. For a brief time after the 1962 publication of Michael Harrington's vivid account of hunger and deprivation, *The Other America,* the consciousness of the nation was awakened. Eventually, however, the political will to reduce poverty was dissipated by the Vietnam War and by a wave of negative reaction to antipoverty programs, which had been oversold and underdeveloped. Yet poverty remained a controversial and festering public issue. The most recent round of debates about poverty was opened in the 1980s as conservative critics turned the tools of social science against liberals, who for a time had held a veritable monopoly on poverty-related research. Prominent among these arguments was *Losing Ground* (1984), in which Charles Murray advanced a cunning argument against government intervention, the thesis that the welfare state was the problem, not the solution, because it promoted dependency and reduced the poor's incentive to work.

Curiously, the controversy surrounding Murray's book may have contributed to the renewal of scholarly interest in poverty. In recent years, social science research has been animated by efforts to reexamine the causes of poverty and the link between welfare programs and long-term disadvantage. Among many social scientists consensus appears to be emerging that government programs play, at most, a trivial role in affecting economic decisions—work and welfare patterns (Bane and Jargowsky 1988). Instead, many experts now believe that, increasingly, poverty can be traced to transformations in the American family. High rates of marital instability and the skyrocketing incidence of out-of-wedlock childbearing are strongly implicated in the growing divisions between rich and poor, especially disparities between advantaged whites and disadvantaged blacks (Garfinkel and McLanahan 1986; Ellwood 1988; Levitan 1988). The recognition of the centrol role of the family in shaping patterns of poverty has prompted researchers to study the specific relationships between family behavior and economic status. This interest extends beyond the experience of single generations to include questions about the extent and nature of intergenerational transmission of poverty—the degree to which impoverishment is passed on from one generation to the next.

These questions are not new. In a report written in the mid-60s, when he was assistant secretary of labor in the Johnson administration, Daniel Patrick Moynihan developed an argument relating family structure and economic disadvantage among blacks (Moynihan 1965). Moynihan reported that high rates of family instability and out-of-wedlock childbearing among blacks created a "tangle of pathology" leading to their disadvantaged economic status. The document was greeted with immense hostility. Moynihan was accused of misreading black culture and blaming the victim (Rainwater and Yancey 1967). However, in the light of recent history, his observations about the black family show prescience. Indeed, contemporary rates of marital disruption and single parenthood make the figures Moynihan cited seem relatively modest by comparison (Cherlin 1992).

There was a spate of social science research in the late 1960s exploring differences between the poor and nonpoor in an effort to answer such questions as: Do the poor have different values? Do they pass these values on to their offspring? And do the values that children acquire early in life substantially affect their prospects of achievement, independent of their parent's social status? These questions were motivated both by the controversy over the Moynihan report and Oscar Lewis's (1959) statements about a "culture of poverty." (See also Banfield 1974.) Extrapolating from his observations of Latin American families, Lewis argued that poor families develop a distinctive code of values and practices that set them apart from the mainstream culture. These attitudes and behaviors are both a response to blocked social opportunities and a further source of entrapment in poverty.

It is not easy to arrive at a summary statement of the results of this vast outpouring of studies (Moynihan 1968; Valentine 1968; Kriesberg 1970; Leacock 1971; Ross and Sawhill 1975). However, at the risk of glossing over some complexities, it is probably fair to say that demonstrating that the poor constitute a distinctive subculture proved to be quite challenging. It was difficult to establish that poor people held very different values of success on such key areas as education, family life, or even psychological propensities such as passivity or deferment of gratification. The modest differences that sometimes emerged from comparisons of poor and nonpoor populations were typically far less conspicuous than the overall pattern of similarity in values, beliefs and even psychological predispositions. Furthermore, evidence that distinctively different attitudes were passed on from parents to children within the family was not terribly impressive. Children adopted values from a variety of sources in addition to parents: the school, mass media, the neighborhood. It could be said that by the mid-1970s, this line of research had died a natural and, some would say, long overdue death. Lewis (1966*a,b*) himself disavowed the validity of a culture of poverty.

However, the debate over the existence of the culture of poverty has now been resurrected in a new form. As part of the justification for cutting back on social welfare programs, growing attention is being given to the rise of the "urban underclass" (Auletta 1983). Once again, the idea is advanced that large numbers of poor people are entrapped in a physical and cultural space that isolates them from mainstream culture. And once again, proponents of this view argue that poor families engage in a range of behaviors that severely compromise their prospects for mobility and social integration. Poor blacks living in areas of concentrated poverty are said to view the world differently and, willingly or reluctantly, adopt an alternative set of goals and behaviors in order to survive the daily demands of life in the ghetto (Stack 1974; Geronimus 1991). These variant standards are thought to be acquired early in life, often within the intimate environment of the family. Growing up in a single-parent household, the offspring of a teen mother, supported by public assistance, is widely believed to prepare a child for a permanent position in the underclass.

Many find a self-perpetuating underclass a compelling idea. Most of the evidence assembled for the existence of an underclass relies on demographic data supplemented with journalistic accounts, but the power of example is enormous (Jencks 1989). In recent years, newspapers and weeklies have been replete with reports graphically describing the breakdown of social order in inner-city urban areas (see, e.g., Dash 1989). These journalistic data have not yet been matched by careful social science research. The term "underclass" has been enthusiastically and, some may say, uncritically adopted in the social science lexicon, often used interchangeably with the "persistently poor." However, not all social scientists have been comfortable with the undifferentiated use of the term "underclass" or the premature conclusion that a growing segment of the urban poor have come to adopt a different set of social values and behaviors. Some have tried to specify the term theoretically, in effect reclaiming its scientific use (Gans 1990).

Most notable among these is William Julius Wilson, who, in *The Truly Disadvantaged* (1987), develops a more general explanation for the growth of the underclass. Wilson links its rise to the erosion of the industrial base in the United States, the decline of well-paying jobs involving heavy labor, the movement of industry out of the urban centers, the flight of middle-class blacks from the ghetto, and the growing social isolation of the most disadvantaged. All of these trends, Wilson argues, have fostered a segment of the poor that is physically and culturally removed from mainstream America. So although Wilson's thesis is rooted in structural changes, he predicts that the growing concentration of the very poor gives rise to a "ghetto-specific culture." Unlike "culture of poverty" theorists, Wilson makes no claim about the autonomy of ghetto culture, but he does argue that situational norms erode the possibility of social mobility.

Wilson's theory is more attractive than earlier formulations because it links macro- and micro-social processes to account for the emergence of the subculture of the urban underclass. But Wilson seems to embrace a rather undifferentiated and overly deterministic view of the individual and family behavior within the ghetto walls. Children born into single-parent families, raised on welfare, and growing up without male supervision are virtually destined to adopt a special worldview that greatly restricts their chances of escaping lifelong poverty. Wilson seems to believe that youth raised in these conditions ultimately perpetuate their disadvantaged circumstances by failing in school, becoming teenage parents, relying on welfare, and rejecting or being rejected by the world of work.

Wilson has bolstered his argument largely with demographic data and ecological associations. In ongoing research, he is also assembling ethnographic and survey data to depict the differences between populations living in areas with high concentrations of poverty. If previous research is any guide, Wilson is likely to establish that individuals growing up in poverty are indeed more likely to manifest problem behavior. Drop-out rates, delinquency, teenage parenthood, idleness will all be higher in areas of concentrated poverty than in areas where poverty levels are lower. Yet, these relative differences in rates of problem behavior conceal another trend that is largely ignored by Wilson and others who focus on broad aggregate comparisons. Despite the popular impression, many children who grow up in poverty, even in poor neighborhoods, find their way out of disadvantage.

In a recent article assessing the strength of the existing literature on the intergenerational transmission of poverty, Duncan and his colleagues (1988) conclude that rather little support exists for the "extent to which welfare dependence is transmitted between generations" or "whether dependence during childhood, either within families or neighborhoods, creates dependence in adulthood." Their analysis from the Michigan Panel on Income Dynamics contradicted the "stereotype of heavy welfare dependency being routinely passed from mother to child" (469). It appears that, at least in the recent past, a good deal of social mobility exists for those who grow up in severely disadvantaged families or who are poor at one point in their lives.

The challenge is, then, to explain the sources of variability in outcomes. How do poor people become assimilated into the mainstream? How do children growing up in poverty escape what so many believe to be the inevitable cycle of disadvantage? These questions are not novel. Students of human development have thought quite a lot about why certain children seem to be "invulnerable" to high-risk situations that might endanger the average disadvantaged child. They have often wondered what is special in the psychological makeup of these so-called resilient children who are able to beat the odds (Werner and Smith 1982; Garmezy and Rutter 1983). As social scientists have begun to look at this question more closely, it has become apparent that protective factors reside not just in the personalities of the children but in the resources available to the children (Furstenberg in press; Sampson 1992). The social environments of poor children are far from identical. Some families are more adaptable, creative, and capable of responding to adversity. Similarly, schools and neighborhoods may be organized in ways that make them more capable of responding to deprivation and danger. To complicate the situation even more, individual children, even within the same kinship, may react to these varied opportunities in contrary ways. So the study of disadvantaged children who do well requires joining the perspectives of sociologists who look at how social environments shape life chances and developmental psychologists who wonder why individuals respond differently to varying social environments.

The Baltimore Study

This chapter describes the preliminary results of an investigation of the extent to which social disadvantage has been inherited and the sources of variation in outcome among a sample of youths who are the off-spring of teenage mothers. As noted above, teenage parenthood is thought by some to be a central link in a cycle of disadvantage; thus children of teenage mothers are a group of particular interest to the study of intergenerational transmission of poverty. The data used here come from an ongoing, twenty-year study of teenage mothers and their children in Baltimore. A principal aim of the Baltimore study has been to identify both conditions that promote the perpetuation of poverty and circumstances that allow disadvantaged persons to enter the economic mainstream.

The Baltimore study has followed the lives of several hundred, mostly black, inner-city women who became pregnant for the first time in the late 1960s. These women were interviewed during pregnancy and at regular intervals for five years thereafter. This portion of the study, completed in 1972, focused on the effect of early childbearing on the life courses of the young mothers, exploring the divergent careers of the teen mothers and a sample of their classmates who postponed childbearing (Furstenberg 1976). After a hiatus of a dozen years, the mothers were reinterviewed in 1983–1984, along with their children, then between the ages of fifteen and seventeen. The seventeen-year follow-up, though it yielded data on both generations, was designed to feature the adults, to assess how the lives of the young mothers changed over time, and to explore sources of variation in their outcomes. In *Adolescent Mothers in Later Life* (1987), which reports the results of the 1984 interviews, the children appear only in a cameo role.

The twenty-year follow-up was intended to give a clear picture of the situation of the next generation. Assessment of their prospects from information in the seventeen-year follow-up was clouded because they were still in the middle of adolescence at that time, a particularly volatile period when life trajectories were not well established. Although the early indications were not encouraging, it was clear from the mothers' experiences that dramatic shifts often occurred over time. Data from the twenty-year follow-up would not only describe the extent to which disadvantage is handed down to the next generation but, when combined with information collected on the youth in early childhood and their mid-teens, would enable a thorough investigation of the sources of a successful transition to adulthood.

The study returned to the field in 1987. This time only a small amount of information was collected from the mothers, largely to provide an independent reading on the situation of the youths. The children of the original group of mothers, now between the ages of eighteen and twenty-one, became the principals in the Baltimore study. An immense amount of information was collected from them in a lengthy interview, a large part of which replicates items contained in the 1988 wave of the National Survey of Children, which permits comparison of the Baltimore youth with a nationally representative sample of comparably aged, black young adults. The Baltimore youth were given a short literacy test to assess where they stand on this critical performance measure. In addition, qualitative case studies of a 10 percent subsample of the respondents were conducted; these data give a more clinical and intimate perspective on the life situations of the respondents.

A word about the sample is in order here. Although it evolved into a longitudinal, multigenerational study, the Baltimore study actually began as an evaluation of one of the first comprehensive care programs for teen mothers in the nation, located at Sinai Hospital in Baltimore. As may be concluded from the origins of the research, most women in the study were black and poor or near-poor. The hospital inevitably drew from its surrounding area, and all the clinic patients received subsidized medical care. Consequently, a high proportion of the sample came from welfare or single-parent families and households with large numbers of children. Most parents were poorly educated and, when they were working, were making modest incomes. Comparisons with health and census data suggested that the women were fairly representative of the larger population of teen mothers, although they may have been a little more diverse than early mothers in the poorest areas of the city.

Over time, the population became a little less diverse. Many of the small number of whites dropped out in the first phase of the study. Whites were more likely to marry, and married women were less likely to stay in the study because of their high rates of mobility. Whites were also more likely to give their children up for adoption. Except for the high rate of attrition among whites and married women in general, there are no obvious strong biases to lead us to suspect that the sample we were able to follow up was very different from the original 400 women in the study. In fact, we did extraordinarily well in retaining subjects. At the seventeen-year follow-up, about 75 percent of the original sample of teen mothers and their children were reinterviewed. In 1987, about 85 percent of the youth who were seen three years earlier were interviewed. In all, close to 70 percent of all eligible black youth in the study are included through the twenty-year follow-up.

Previous Results

It is too early to provide more than a descriptive account of some early impressions of the twenty-year follow-up. But some of these preliminary findings are intriguing. Before we describe them, it will be useful to begin by briefly summarizing what was already known before this recent round of data collection began.

The family circumstances of the Baltimore children were far from ideal at the time they were born. Almost all of their mothers were still in high school or had already dropped out before their babies' birth. Only a fifth of their parents were married by the time they were born. Most spent their infancy in the households of their grandparents, who were generally uneducated and impoverished. The situation of the children at birth did not present a very encouraging picture.

And this picture did not greatly improve in the early part of the study. Their preschool years were characterized by a great deal of flux. Many of their parents married, but close to half of the marriages broke up by the time of the five-year folllow-up in 1972. The majority of the children had some contact with their fathers, but as the study progressed, paternal participation became more fleeting and episodic. As new households were formed and then dissolved, the children were sometimes put in the care of their grandparents or other relatives.

Relatives, usually the maternal grandmother, were often called upon to help out as the young mothers struggled to establish a toehold in the labor market. About two-thirds of the families relied on public assistance while the young mothers tried to complete high school or find stable employment. Family life was further complicated as many of the young mothers had second and even third children in their late teens and early twenties.

On the brighter side, most of the children experienced normal deliveries and had few serious health problems during infancy and their preschool years. In 1972, the children were given a series of developmental tests, and assessments of the children were gathered from the parents. As well as could be determined, the vast majority of the children were not exhibiting behavioral abnormalities. They performed normally on the Peabody Picture Vocabulary Test, at least by comparison with other urban black youth, and from the parents' reports, serious developmental difficulties were detected in only a small minority of cases.

The information collected in 1984 allows reconstruction of portions of the later childhood of the youth in the study with some confidence, although there are some important gaps. The mothers' lives seemed to stabilize over time. Over two-thirds were able to complete high school, find employment, and get off public assistance. By the seventeen-year follow-up, only a quarter were on welfare; another quarter were working poor; the rest were evenly divided between those with modest incomes and the lucky minority who were able to make it into the middle class. Nearly all of the middle-class group were among the 38 percent of the women who were married in 1984. Even within that select subgroup, only half had been in stable marriages. Just one woman in six was living with the father of her child.

Despite considerable marital instability, relatively few women went on to have additional children after their early twenties. By 1984, only 12 percent had had any additional childrn in the preceding five years. Many who became pregnant a third or fourth time obtained abortions, and eventually more than half of the women sought sterilization, even although they were still in the prime of their childbearing years.

So the situation of the children was more economically secure by 1984, but only a tiny fraction had experienced what could be called a reasonably stable childhood. Few resided with their father continuously. Among those that did not, most saw their fathers only occasionally or not at all. Only a sixth of the children—a fifth of those not living with their fathers—saw them as often as once a week on the average.

Most youth were, however, living with their mothers and had done so continuously throughout the study. Still, one in four had experienced a separation lasting more than three months, and a tenth had been apart from them for at least two years. Quite a substantial number of these children had lived with their maternal grandmothers at some time during the study. Varied family experiences were common. A third of the children claimed to have persons who were like mothers to them other than their biological mothers. This acknowledgment did not necessarily mean that their own mothers were not their primary caretakers. Both the data collected early in the study and in the 1984 interview revealed that most of the children had been raised primarily by their biological mothers (Fursternberg and Harris 1990).

A wide array of indicators of well-being were collected on the youth in 1984—how they were doing in school, getting along with family members and with their peers, prosocial and delinquent activities, and their emotional health. For the purposes of comparison, the well-being of the Baltimore youth was compared to that of their counterparts in the 1981 National Survey of Children. Because there were so few whites in the Baltimore sample by 1984, the comparisons are confined to black youth. Considering the very small numbers involved, there is impressive similarity across a wide array of indicators between the offspring of young

TABLE 7.1

Behavior of Black Youths Ages 15 and 16, Baltimore Study, 1984, and
National Survey of Children, 1981

	BALTIMORE STUDY (%)	NSC: MOTHER'S FIRST BIRTH AT AGE 17 OR LESS (%)	NSC: MOTHER'S FIRST BIRTH AT AGE 20 OR OVER (%)
Class standing above average	26	31	31
Ever repeated a grade	53	46	17
Skipped school, last year	29	27	14
Fought at school, last year	28	39	15
Damaged school property, last year	3	15	2
Parents received note from school about behavior, last 5 years	56	55	15
Parents brought to school about behavior, last 5 years	41	42	17
Suspended/expelled, last 5 years	49	36	19
Stayed out too late, last year	74	76	67
Lied to parents about something important, last year	56	52	39
Stole something, last year	10	18	6
Hurt someone seriously, last year	16	9	15
Ever ran away from home	23	6	0
Ever stopped by police	33	27	9
Ever drank alcohol	54	42	44
Got drunk, last year	21	18	10
Ever smoked pot	44	24	25
Ever tried other drugs	4	3	0
Ever had sex	78	58	35
Ever been pregnant	11	15	2
N	202	33	52

mothers in the local sample when compared to a nationally representative one (see table 7.1).

No less impressive is the magnitude of the differences between the offspring of black early and later childbearers, though surely some of these differences cannot be causally linked to the timing of the first birth but reflect dissimilar endowments and fertility backgrounds. On many of the indicators, the children of mothers who postponed parenthood outperform the children of teen mothers by a wide margin; on almost all, differences between the two groups occur in the predicted direction. The study confirms what everyone suspected—having a teenage mother is associated with problem behavior in middle adolescence. However, a sizable fraction were doing reasonably well in 1984.

In accounting for this variation, the analysis was able to show that the problems experienced by the children could be linked directly to the mothers' experiences in managing the transition to adulthood. As the mothers' lives changed over time for the better or worse, often, though not invariably, their children's behavior improved or deteriorated accordingly. It would be misleading to overstate the degree of correspondence in the trajectories of mother and child. In fact, the effects were quite complex, making it difficult to detect recurring patterns. For example, the children of mothers who moved off welfare during the study were much less likely to experience grade failure than those whose parents continued to receive public assistance or who initiated a spell of welfare later in the study. Similarly, children reaped benefits in school performance when their mothers improved their educational status during the study. In contrast, early additional fertility produced lasting school problems for children that were not offset in the later years of the study. Moreover, these same events in the mother's lives did not produce uniform results in other outcomes, such as delinquency or substance abuse.

That fluidity and flexibility in the mother's life course forecasts change in the child's circumstances is a happy finding for policymakers. But, if these data provide any guide, researchers are going to be hard put to predict just what kinds of events will predict what kinds of outcomes for which children.

Preliminary Findings
from the Twenty-Year Follow-up

The twenty-year follow-up is intended to further explore the intriguing and largely unexplored question of how children's lives are affected by the changing circumstances of their parents' lives. But the scope of inquiry has been expanded to include other changes in the youths' environment—school, the neighborhood—and how they shape the transition to early adulthood. To make these questions more manageable, the present analysis will concentrate on a relatively small number of indicators of well-being, just as did the analysis of the changing life courses of the original mothers. This chapter, based on very preliminary results of only a portion of the data that are being assembled, gives some flavor of what is expected from more extensive analysis.

The youth in 1987 are on average nineteen, just a shade over three years older than when last seen. Now that there is a fairly complete record of their teen years, it is possible to report on two key milestones— whether they completed high school, and whether they avoided premature parenthood. These critical markers of a successful transition to early adulthood are presented in table 7.2, along with a host of related indicators of well-being. These measures are shown by age, as not all the Baltimore youth have reached the end of their teens and some of these measures are age sensitive.

Some progression by age is evident both in the positive as well as the negative indicators of well-being. The older youth are more likely to have graduated from high school, entered the labor market, and earned more than $10,000 in the previous year. They are also more likely to have had a live birth, committed a serious property offense, and been in jail. Many of the measures tapping school performance, substance abuse, and mental health are unrelated to age.

The 1984 interview revealed marked differences in behavior among males and females, especially in school achievement and deviant behavior. The same pattern shows up three years later, as can be seen in table 7.3, which shows these same indicators by gender. Males are much more likely to have repeated a grade and dropped out of school. The disparity in educational attainment is somewhat lower because more females have become parents, leading to a delay in high school graduation. Still, two-thirds of the females have graduated or obtained a GED, compared to 57 percent of the males. Males and females are equally likely to be employed, however. Sharp differences by gender exist on almost all the measures of deviant behavior, with males reporting levels far above those of females. An extraordinarily high proportion of males have had encounters with the police and have been in jail. As in the analysis of the 1984 data, it is possible to compare the status of the Baltimore youth with the situation of their counterparts in the National Survey of Children, this time the 1988 version of the NSC. Table 7.4 shows the same set of indicators for black youth aged eighteen through twenty-one in the 1988 National Survey of children, weighted to be nationally representative. The outcomes are also shown by mother's age at first birth. The youth whose mothers were seventeen or younger at their first birth match the Baltimore sample, while the offspring of the later childbearers

TABLE 7.2

Youths Who Have Experienced Selected Events, by Age, Baltimore Study, 1987

		AGE		
	TOTAL (%)	18 (%)	19 (%)	20–21 (%)
Graduated from high school	62.7	42.9	63.1	69.5
In school	37.3	54.3	37.7	30.5
Ever dropped out of HS	34.4	31.4	35.2	34.4
Ever repeated a grade	42.4	54.3	43.4	36.8
Currently married	4.0	5.7	1.6	6.3
Living with partner	6.0	11.0	5.7	4.2
Had sex	96.4	94.3	97.5	95.7
Ever pregnant	49.2	34.3	48.4	55.8
Had live birth	31.3	20.0	32.0	34.7
Currently employed	56.3	40.4	55.7	63.2
Welfare in 1986	12.0	11.4	14.9	8.4
Annual income				
less than $5,000	65.6	71.5	72.5	54.7
$5,000–$9,999	20.4	22.9	18.3	22.1
$10,000 and over	12.4	2.9	9.2	20.0
Ever suspended/expelled	54.6	68.6	50.4	54.7
Ever used pot	57.5	57.1	54.1	62.1
Ever used cocaine	13.1	17.1	8.2	17.9
Ever damaged property	27.4	28.6	22.1	33.7
Ever carried hidden weapon	15.5	11.4	13.1	20.0
Ever stolen item worth $50+	9.9	5.7	8.2	13.7
Ever attacked person to hurt	12.3	20.0	6.6	16.8
Ever sold drugs	14.3	8.6	10.7	21.1
Ever stopped by police	46.8	48.6	43.4	50.5
Ever been in jail	16.3	8.6	13.1	23.2
Think life going very well	31.3	34.3	35.2	25.3
N	252	35	122	95

provide a baseline against which to judge the accomplishments of the Baltimore youth.

The correspondence between the youth in the Baltimore study and in the NSC is mixed. On many of the measures the Baltimore youth do not diverge remarkably from the national sample of children of young mothers. Notable exceptions, however, are the education measures, and employment and welfare measures, and a few of the delinquency measures,

TABLE 7.3

Youths Who Have Experienced Selected Events, by Gender, Baltimore Study, 1987

| | | GENDER | |
	TOTAL (%)	MALE (%)	FEMALE (%)
Graduated from high school	62.7	57.6	67.7
In school	37.3	35.2	39.4
Ever dropped out of HS	34.4	39.8	29.1
Ever repeated a grade	42.4	48.8	36.2
Currently married	4.0	1.6	6.3
Living with partner	6.0	1.6	10.2
Had sex	96.4	97.6	95.2
Ever pregnant	49.2	41.6	56.7
Had live birth	31.3	24.8	37.8
Currently employed	56.3	58.4	54.3
Welfare in 1986	12.0	0	23.8
Annual income			
Less than $5,000	65.6	63.2	68.0
$5,000–$9,999	20.4	20.0	20.8
$10,000 and over	12.4	15.2	9.6
Ever suspended/expelled	54.6	67.7	41.7
Ever used pot	57.5	66.4	48.8
Ever used cocaine	13.1	19.2	7.1
Ever damaged property	27.4	40.0	15.0
Ever carried hidden weapon	15.5	26.4	4.7
Ever stolen item worth $50+	9.9	17.6	2.4
Ever attacked person to hurt	12.3	15.2	9.4
Ever sold drugs	14.3	24.0	4.7
Ever stopped by police	46.8	75.0	19.0
Ever been in jail	16.3	30.4	2.4
Think life going very well	31.3	28.0	34.6
N	252	125	127

on which the Baltimore youth are worse off. It is likely that some of this divergence is due to the largely urban character of the Baltimore sample. A further source of divergence is in the character of the surveys themselves, the most important among these being the season in which the interviews were conducted. The Baltimore study was conducted in the spring and summer, while the NSC was done in the fall and winter.

TABLE 7.4

Black Youths Aged 18–21 Who Have Experienced Selected Events, by Age of Mother at First Birth, National Survey of Children, 1988

	TOTAL (%)	MOTHER'S FIRST BIRTH AT AGE 17 OR LESS (%)	MOTHER'S FIRST BIRTH AT AGE 20 OR OVER (%)
Graduated from high school	85.8	82.4	88.9
In school	37.4	22.8	55.2
Ever dropped out of HS	17.3	21.3	12.2
Ever repeated a grade	26.4	28.4	21.8
Currently married	7.8	6.8	12.0
Living with partner	7.0	6.7	2.8
Had sex	87.0	92.0	95.6
Ever pregnant	35.6	45.9	28.0
Had live birth	27.6	35.5	19.1
Currently employed	63.5	45.1	64.9
Welfare in last year	14.8	24.6	10.7
Annual income			
Less than $5,000	71.9	71.9	70.0
$5,000–$9,999	10.6	7.3	15.0
$10,000 and over	17.5	20.8	15.0
Ever suspended/expelled	42.6	59.0	29.8
Ever used pot	46.3	55.4	44.6
Ever used cocaine	7.2	8.7	10.7
Ever damaged property	19.1	33.4	13.4
Ever carried hidden weapon	7.9	8.8	5.5
Ever stolen item worth $50+	4.3	12.2	.9
Ever attacked person to hurt	6.4	2.9	11.8
Ever sold drugs	7.4	14.6	3.7
Ever stopped by police	27.4	30.6	28.0
Ever been in jail	1.8	3.1	.8
Think life going very well	41.9	28.3	47.9
Base N	174	57	68

Note: Observations weighted to make sample nationally representative. Cases with mother's age at first birth 18 or 19 included in total column.

This could contribute to the large differences in high school graduation, school enrollment, and, perhaps, employment.

Despite the differences between Baltimore's children and those of early childbearers in the NSC, both are uniformly worse off than the children of later childbearers in the NSC. On nearly all of the measures, the difference is in the expected direction; in many cases the difference is quite large.

In these tables, there is little to lead to a revision of the earlier conclusion: a substantial minority of youths born to teenage mothers are experiencing severe difficulties in managing the transition to adulthood. Even so, these findings must be put in perspective. A large proportion of the youth in the Baltimore sample grew up in the so-called underclass. Given all the handicaps accrued during childhood—starting out life as the offspring of young and usually unmarried mothers, encountering bouts of severe and extended poverty, growing up under uncertain and changing family situations, and provided with only limited contact and support from their biological fathers—it is perhaps remarkable that so many of the Baltimore youth give signs of finding their way out of disadvantage. While the Baltimore youth are not so well off as the children of later childbearers, it is clear that the majority are experiencing successful transitions to adulthood.

This variation in results is impressive. It is a finding that challenges both social scientists and policymakers to search for the conditions within the individual, family, school, and neighborhood that explain the sources of resilience. By all accounts, many of these youth are indeed "beating the odds." How do they do it?

As a start on an answer to this important question, two indicators from the array in tables 7.2 and 7.3 were selected as general indications of a successful transition to adulthood. The first is whether the teen had a child before age nineteen. This measure can be constructed for everyone except the small number of eighteen-year-olds, who were counted as parents if they were pregnant at the time of the interview.

The other measure involved a little more computation. It is a combined measure of educational and occupational attainment, a variant of socioeconomic status. In the highest category are high school graduates now attending college; next come graduates who are currently employed but no longer in school; the third category are youth in transition from school into the labor force (some of whom have graduated but are looking for work) and youth still in school; the fourth category are high school dropouts looking for work or attending job training programs; the bottom group are those drop-outs who are unemployed and not looking for work. Slightly less than half of the Baltimore youth fall in the top two categories, and about a third are in the bottom two. The younger youth in the study are predictably more often assigned to the middle category because some of them have not yet had time to complete high school. This creates only a minor problem because of their small number.

The measure of attainment was constructed to take into account dropping out of high school, so that we know that those in the bottom categories invariably have a history of dropping out of school. Still, it is surprising to discover how few youth in the top three categories ever left school before graduating. Similarly, we discovered huge differences in the frequency of early childbearing, that is parenthood before age nineteen, by attainment status. The high achievers rarely become parents, and the low achievers often do. The differences among males are not so sharp but are still quite evident. On the other hand, males with low attainment are much more likely to have criminal records.

Figure 7.1 shows that this measure of economic attainment is a remarkably sensitive indicator of the youth's integration into mainstream society as measured by various signs of economic success: whether the youth has a savings or checking account, a credit card, a driver's license, or a vehicle. These are signs of making it in American society. Having a driver's license and a car undoubtedly also improves the chances of employment. Indeed, as could be anticipated, youth in the top two categories were about twice as likely to have paid taxes as in the bottom two. Even so, note that close to half of the youth in the fourth category had paid taxes in the preceding year, suggesting that many of these young adults are struggling to enter the labor force.

The youth in the study were asked to rate their contentment with various features of their lives. Figure 7.2 charts the extent to which they reported wanting to change selected dimensions of their lives by the measure of economic achievement. The measure of attainment tracks extremely well how the youth feel they are doing and how they are feeling about themselves.

These results are persuasive that this measure of attainment is an appropriate way of capturing in a single, global indicator an important dimension of the economic transition to adulthood. Youth at the top are making it. Youth at the bottom are not. Moreover, those at the top generally feel good about themselves, and those at the bottom, not surprisingly, are more often discontented.

A similar analysis examining those who have become teen parents generally shows the same patterns, but they are far less pronounced. Teen parents are not doing so well economically. Self-ratings indicated that they are less content with their lives. But when their lower economic status is taken into account, teen parenthood does not produce life dissatisfaction in the same way that lower educational and economic attainment do. In fact, it may contribute to greater satisfaction. Still, many teen parents are less than happy about their life circumstances— even the fact that they are parents so early in life.

FIGURE 7.1

Selected Correlates of Transition to Adulthood, by Attainment Group,
Baltimore Study, 1987

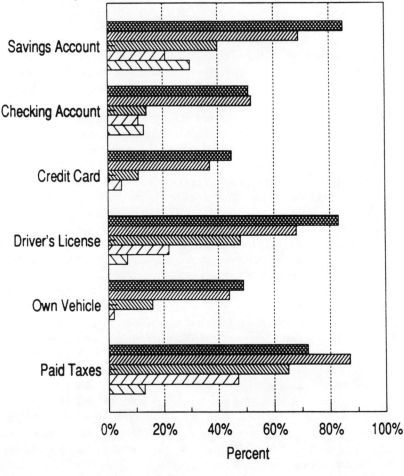

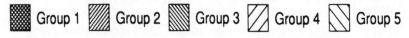

Now it is time to address the question that has prompted the continuation of the Baltimore study: why are some youth who grow up in disadvantaged circumstances managing the transition to adulthood successfully while others are not? Again, the results presented here are based on a very preliminary inspection of the data, but they hint at what is

FIGURE 7.2

How Much Respondent Would Like to Change Various Aspects of His or Her Life, by Attainment Group, Baltimore Study, 1987

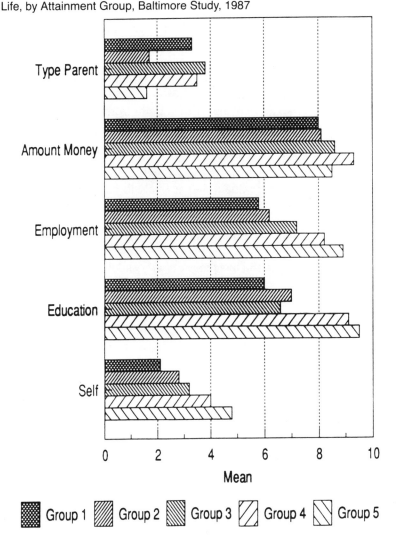

likely to be discovered. The aim is to elaborate the model built in our *Adolescent Mothers in Later Life* (1987), which examined how children's changing family circumstances altered their chances of successful adjustment, this time also linking change in the neighborhood and school contexts to the course of development in the child's lives.

A first step to this ambitious plan is to examine some of the precursors to a successful transition to adulthood as measured by economic attainment and avoidance of early parenthood. It is already apparent that, although these two outcomes are connected, they are not necessarily the result of similar kinds of socializing experiences. Further, the pathways to success for males and females may very well be different. The precursors selected for consideration here are two central circumstances in the children's lives: the stability of their family life from birth to adolescence and whether they grew up on public assistance. Patterns of marital disruption and welfare experience provide a point from which to examine how children's changing family environments affect their life chances.

At first glance, it appears that there is only a modest association between the children's family situation during adolescence and their ability to negotiate the transition to adulthood. Children whose mothers were married in 1984 were about half as likely to be in the bottom two categories of our attainment measure as those whose parents had never married and about a third as likely as those whose parents were separated or divorced. On the other hand, no differences occur by marital status of the mothers in the top two categories. And there were no significant differences in the incidence of early childbearing by mothers' marital status. This finding did not change when the currently married were divided by whether they were in first marriages or subsequent ones.

That the marital status of the parents seemed to have such a small effect on high achievement and avoidance of early childbearing was surprising. Existing theory and research leads suggest that children will fare better in stable family environments. Could remarriage be making up for early bouts of instability? A closer look at the data suggests that the theory is not misguided. A different sorting of marriages produces quite different results.

We compared children in three types of marital situations: those who spent their entire childhood with their biological fathers in the home; children who spent at least ten years living with their biological fathers or stepfather and were still living with them in 1984; and children whose mothers married later in the study but were still married in 1984. The numbers are small, but the findings are suggestive. Children in recently remarried households clearly do worse than those who have spent most of their lives in a two-parent household. There is little evidence based on these particular outcomes that marriage to the biological father was critical to the child's successful transition to adulthood. If anything, youth were a little better off if their mothers waited to marry, probably because the women who waited to wed more often completed school.

TABLE 7.5

Distribution across Attainment Groups and Percent Having Early Birth, by Mother's Welfare Experience through 1984, Baltimore Study, 1987

	WELFARE EXPERIENCE				
	never on welfare (%)	short past (%)	short recent (%)	long past (%)	long recent (%)
Attainment group					
1	30.3	21.8	11.1	13.2	4.9
2	30.3	21.8	22.2	29.0	19.5
3	22.7	25.4	25.9	21.1	24.4
4	10.6	21.8	29.6	26.3	26.8
5	6.1	9.1	11.1	10.5	24.4
Early birth	13.6	18.2	18.5	34.2	41.5
N	66	55	27	38	41

Interestingly, children of the more recently married women actually were as likely to be low achievers and become teenage parents as youth whose parents were divorced or never married.

Thus, marital decisions of the mothers are implicated in the children's pattern of success. But, if the Baltimore results are any basis for generalization, the relationship between marital careers and children's success in later life may not be a simple one. How is marital stability translated into developmental advantage? Marital continuity must have payoff for children beyond the provision of resources. Otherwise one marriage would be as good as another. One reason may be that children in longstanding relationships are more likely to form deep and enduring ties with their fathers or stepfathers, and men in these circumstances play a protective role in the children's lives. These speculations move beyond the results, but it will be possible to look at relevant bits of evidence in further analysis (Furstenberg and Harris 1990).

The 1984 data showed that, like marital experience, mothers' experiences on welfare profoundly affected their children's life chances. Certainly this finding should not come as a surprise to anyone. It is less clear why and how growing up on welfare creates a lasting disadvantage for children. Consider the evidence in table 7.5, showing how mothers' welfare experience through 1984 is related to the youths' likelihood of economic success and postponement of childbearing at the twenty-year follow-up. The more years a mother spent on welfare, the lower the achievement of her child and the higher the risk of premature parenthood. Table 7.5 also shows how the life chances of the children are affected when parents exit from welfare. Any welfare experience, whether long or short, in the distant or recent past, reduces a youth's chances of educational and economic success. A long history of welfare, on the other hand, appears not to greatly affect a youth's chances of entering parenthood at an early age so long as the welfare spell ended by 1984. It looks as if only persistent and continuous welfare experience increases the odds of early childbearing. This finding is an intriguing reminder of what was learned from the earlier analysis. Events in the mothers' lives may affect the children's outcomes differently depending on the timing of the events and the type of outcome. However, the numbers are small, so the findings are only suggestive.

Knowing that welfare experience reduces a child's economic prospects is hardly a revelation. The challenge for researchers is to say why. For example, are children worse off growing up on welfare than they would be if their families were poor but did not receive public assistance? A long history of welfare does seem to carry greater risk of prospective disadvantage in the next generation. The children of working poor single mothers score much higher on the measure of attainment than the offspring of chronic welfare mothers. And they are less prone to early childbearing as well.

Of course these two groups—families on welfare and the working poor—are not completely comparable. Those women who are persistently on welfare undoubtedly have less education and fewer marketable skills. They have larger families and more crowded households, they may be more depressed and discontented with their lives, they may live in more distressed neighborhoods, and their children may have attended worse schools. In short, being chronically on welfare carries a host of risk factors that compromise their children's life chances.

It must also be remembered that a substantial minority of the youth who spent most or all of their childhood on welfare and were still on welfare in 1984 appear to be escaping from poverty in 1987. A quarter have graduated from high school and another quarter are still in school; and 45 percent of the girls and 71 percent of the boys (59 percent of all youth who grew up on welfare) did not become parents before age nineteen. We must be able to explain these "deviant" cases as well as to pinpoint how long-term welfare experience produces such detrimental effects on the life chances of youth. This involves a much more detailed study than anyone has yet provided of how the discrete risks associated with growing up on welfare (marital instability, limited resources, schooling, neighborhood) contribute to a youth's problems of making it out of poverty.

Conclusion

This chapter is a downpayment, and not a very large one at that, for a future analysis that maps the prominent routes out of poverty for children who grow up in disadvantaged families.

Thus far we know that, like their mothers, the lives of the youth in the Baltimore study are becoming more varied over time. By early adulthood, many show the earmarks of success; some are struggling to get a toehold in the middle class; and, a substantial minority are not faring well at all. Given the circumstances of their birth, it is impressive that two-thirds have completed high school or got a GED or are close to doing so. Three-quarters had not had a birth before age nineteen—85 percent of the males and 64 percent of the females. But a third of the youth have dropped out of school, and many of these young adults are unemployable. A third of the males have spent time in jail, and more than one in ten of the older youth are currently incarcerated.

We have learned from the Baltimore study that the cycle of poverty and disadvantage is neither inevitable nor even typical. But the transmission of disadvantage is common enough to justify the concern of policymakers. If we are to be effective in targeting services for the "truly disadvantaged," we must have a clearer understanding of how disadvantage compromises a child's life chances. If we know why many youth navigate their way out of poverty, we may be in better position to help those who cannot. Is it because their needs are greater, their resources less, or are they simply less fortunate in finding the escape routes out of poverty? Academic research has made only a small start in addressing these critical questions. They should be at the top of our research agenda in the decade ahead.

NOTE

This research was supported by grants from the Ford and Robert Wood Johnson Foundations, and written while Furstenberg and Brooks-Gunn were fellows at the Russell Sage Foundation. The chapter benefited from useful coments by Marta Tienda.

MARIS A. VINOVSKIS

8 Historical Perspectives on Adolescent Pregnancy

Problems associated with adolescent sexuality, pregnancy, and childbearing continue to preoccupy the American public and policymakers. Yet most discussions of these issues concentrate on the present. This is unfortunate because it limits our ability to place these concerns in a broader, historical perspective that could help to explain how and why this set of issues emerged in the last fifteen years as one of the major domestic priorities for the federal government.

Rather than attempt to provide a comprehensive historical survey of adolescent pregnancy, this chapter will examine three specific topics: (1) adolescent pregnancy in colonial and nineteenth-century America; (2) the recent "epidemic" of adolescent pregnancy; and (3) the struggle over the definition of the problem of adolescent pregnancy. Particular attention is paid to the prolonged dependency of youth as well as the increased burden of welfare dependency and "opportunity costs" for the young, unmarried mother today. While these topics by no means exhaust the issue historically, they will at least illustrate how one may view adolescent pregnancy from a broader perspective.

Adolescent Sexuality, Pregnancy, and Childbearing in Colonial and Nineteenth-Century America

Adolescent sexuality, pregnancy, and childbearing are viewed by many today as serious problems, but colonial and nineteenth-century Americans were not as concerned (Vinovskis 1986a). Neither have the few historians of adolescence (Kett 1977) paid much attention to these matters; nor have those who study fertility trends in the past (Vinovskis 1981; Wells 1985).

One of the popular explanations why adolescent pregnancy was not important in early America is that the age of menarche in the past was much higher than today, so that few teenage women were mature enough biologically to become pregnant. Indeed, one estimate suggests that the age of menarche for some European women in the early nineteenth century was as high as seventeen or eighteen years (Wyshak and Frisch 1982).

We do not have firm data on the age of menarche for women in early America. Studies of the nineteenth century suggest that the age of menarche was about fifteen in the United States in the late nineteenth century (Wyshak and Frisch 1982). Since the onset of menarche is related to nutrition, one can speculate that the age of menarche was about fifteen or sixteen in early America because colonial Americans were similar to their nineteenth-century counterparts in stature and nutrition (Frisch and McArthur 1974; Jones 1980; Fogel 1986). Therefore, the lack of concern about adolescent pregnancy in early America cannot be explained simply by the biological differences between our ancestors and ourselves.

If most colonial American women married as young teenagers, then the problems associated with adolescent childbearing today may not have seemed as serious when everyone was marrying at an early age. Most scholars in the late nineteenth and early twentieth centuries believed that colonial New England women married and had children as young teenagers (Earle 1895; Calhoun 1960). More recent scholarship, however, demonstrates that relatively few women in colonial New England married or had children as young adolescents (Demos 1970; Greven 1970; Lockridge 1970). Most women married in their early twenties, and the age at first marriage for both women and men rose in the nineteenth century (Vinovskis 1981). As a result, only 3.6 percent of native-born women and 4.7 percent of foreign-born women ages fourteen to nineteen in Massachusetts were married in the late nineteenth century (Massachusetts 1887). In the early twentieth century there was a shift toward younger marriages, with a low point in the median age of marriage reached in the 1950s (Vinovskis 1988c).

If biological or nuptial explanations cannot account for the lack of attention to adolescent pregnancy earlier, perhaps the answer may be that society in the past so thoroughly controlled the sexual behavior of young single people that premarital pregnancies rarely occurred. After all, the traditional image of the New England Puritans is one of very strict and repressive attitudes toward sex in general.

Again, historians suggest a much more complex view of sexuality among early Americans. The Puritans were not reluctant to discuss or enjoy sex; they were only unwilling to tolerate premarital or extramarital sex (Morgan 1966; Degler 1980). In addition, the strong social sanctions against premarital sex in New England lasted only from about 1630 to 1660 (Thompson 1986). Thereafter, despite the continued injunctions of Puritan ministers, New England couples increasingly engaged in premarital sex after becoming engaged (Hindus and Smith 1975; Tracy 1979). In fact, the practice of bundling, where an unmarried couple with their clothes on slept in the same bed, became popular in the early eighteenth century (Stiles 1934).

The shift in attitudes toward premarital sex was reflected in changes in the rate of premaritally conceived first births. From a low rate of less than 10 percent in the seventeenth century, it rose to nearly 30 percent in the second half of the eighteenth century (Hindus and Smith 1975). Thus, our ancestors were not always hostile to any premarital sex. Acceptable premarital sex, however, was not associated with casual dating but confined mainly to couples already planning to get married or formally engaged (Vinovskis 1988a).

During the early nineteenth century, there was a substantial decrease in premaritally conceived births, so that by the time of the Civil War sexual intercourse was no longer viewed as a normal or tolerated component of the courtship process. This dramatic reversal reflected the efforts of early nineteenth-century reformers, as part of the Second Great Awakening, to emphasize that any premarital sexual activity was sinful and wrong (Juster 1988). The negative view of premarital sex was reinforced by the medical community, which now argued that any early sexual activity was dangerous to the physical development of adolescents (Alcott 1856). Finally, the prohibition against premarital sex was strengthened by the idea of the "fallen woman" that viewed women who had experienced premarital sexual intercourse as unfit for marriage (Berg 1978).

Rather than seeing the recent increases in adolescent sexual activity as unusual, one may view them as part of the broader, long-term fluctuations in sexual behavior. Those who argue that high rates of premarital sexual activity cannot be reversed are incorrect from a historical perspective, since both European and American societies experienced great changes in premarital sexual activity over time (Laslett et al. 1980). Whether the same social mechanism for reducing premarital sexual activity in the past could or should be employed today is less clear. The type of severe, negative sanctions applied earlier, particularly to single women, to discourage early sexual activity probably is neither ethically nor politically permissible in most of our society today. Therefore, the question remains: What types of arguments, positive inducements, or mild negative disincentives can be used to persuade teenagers today to postpone early sexual activity and whether these efforts can really be very effective?

As American society witnessed great changes in the overall rate of premaritally conceived first births in the seventeenth, eighteenth, and nineteenth centuries, were adolescents singled out as a group in need of special attention or assistance? Rarely, because early Americans did not view adolescence as a relatively separate and distinct phase of the life course until the late nineteenth and early twentieth centuries (Demos and Demos 1969; Juster and Vinovskis 1987). Whenever there was concern about practices such as premarital sex or intemperance, it was directed toward that behavior in general throughout the entire population rather than on a particular age-group such as teenagers.

Adolescent pregnancy and early childbearing within the context of an economically viable marriage were not deemed a social problem in early America because there was little visible evidence that the individuals involved suffered any great or permanent damage. While everyone was expected to receive a common school education by the mid-nineteenth century, most students completed their schooling by age fifteen or sixteen anyway (Cremin 1980; Kaestle and Vinovskis 1980). Since married women were expected to stay at home, an early marriage was not seen as disrupting any long-term career plans or opportunities (Mason et al. 1978; Degler 1980). Furthermore, since few couples ever divorced, no particular risk of marital disruption was associated with an adolescent pregnancy and marriage (Griswold 1982). Thus, although few nineteenth-century writers and parents actually encouraged adolescent marriages and childbearing, if they did occur they were not regarded as a calamity as long as the young couple could support themselves without any private or public charity.

An "Epidemic" of Adolescent Pregnancy?

From time to time local groups dealt with aspects of the problem of adolescent pregnancy during the twentieth century. Juvenile courts were established in the early twentieth century in part to deal with young, unmarried girls who became sexually active (Schlossman and Wallach 1980). Homes for unwed pregnant adolescents were established with the expectation that most of these mothers would put their children up for adoption (Brumberg 1985). But it was only in the second half of the 1970s that the mass media and the federal government suddenly seemed to discover adolescent pregnancy as a major national problem necessitating immediate federal intervention. Indeed, the secretary of the Department of Health and Human Services in 1978 proclaimed adolescent pregnancy as one of the top domestic problems of the Carter administration in 1978 (Vinovskis 1988a).

To dramatize the problem, the media and policymakers in Washington referred to an "epidemic" of adolescent pregnancy. While "epidemic" was not always clearly specified, most commentators implied that the rate of adolescent pregnancy was at an unprecedented high and threatened the well-being of the next generation.

But was there an unprecedented epidemic of adolescent pregnancy in the late 1970s? If one looks at the rate of adolescent childbearing, for which we have good data, it had peaked twenty years earlier. The rate of teenage childbearing increased sharply after World War II and reached a peak of 97.3 births per 1,000 women ages fifteen to nineteen in 1957. At the time when the epidemic of adolescent pregnancy was stressed in Washington in 1977, the rate of fertility had declined to 52.8 births per 1,000 women ages 15–19 and had by 1983 leveled off at 51.7 births. Although the legalization of abortions in 1973 helped to maintain a relatively low rate of teenage childbearing, given the estimated increases in the rate of teenage pregnancies during the 1970s, the overall rate of adolescent pregnancy was still lower than in 1957 (Vinovskis 1988a). Thus, if the simple demographics of adolescent pregnancy and childbearing had determined social policy, the federal programs for teenagers should have been enacted during the Eisenhower administration.

If the so-called epidemic of adolescent pregnancy occurred two decades earlier, why was this problem suddenly discovered and publicized in the mid-1970s? There are several factors that contributed. During the 1950s it was not unusual for even adult women to experience an unintended pregnancy because reliable and effective contraceptives such as the pill were still unavailable (U.S. Congress, House, Select Committee on Population 1978). In addition, the legal barriers to providing contraceptive services, especially to unmarried teenagers, made it unlikely that many individuals or groups would attempt to distribute such information or devices (Dienes 1972; Reed 1983). Only in the late 1960s and early 1970s, with the legalization (by court decisions) of contraceptive services, did it become easy to provide family planning services to large numbers of sexually active teenagers (Hayes 1987).

Adolescent pregnancy did not appear to be a major social problem in the 1950s because most pregnant teenagers quickly and quietly married the father (Chase-Lansdale and Vinovskis 1987). As a result, the welfare costs associated with adolescent pregnancies were much lower than two decades later when the population and number of out-of-wedlock births had increased dramatically and the amount of welfare benefits available to single mothers had increased substantially (Garfinkel and McLanahan 1986).

The expectations and opportunities for young women had also improved since the 1950s. Whereas policymakers in the 1950s assumed that most women would get married and stay at home to raise their children, by the 1970s it was apparent that many of these women would also pursue a career (Gatlin 1987; Mintz and Kellogg 1988). The increasing rate of divorce also suggested that many women who were married would have to support themselves as single women later in their lives (Weitzman 1985). Furthermore, the expectation and need for more education in order to obtain a good job increased. As a result, dropping out of school because of an unintended adolescent pregnancy was now seen as a more serious handicap for these women and their infants than ever before.

Behind much of the concern about adolescent pregnancy and early childbearing during the 1970s was the question of abortion. With the legalization of abortion by the Supreme Court in 1973, both "pro-life" and "pro-choice" legislators sought ways of diffusing this issue indirectly through other legislation (Jackson and Vinovskis 1983). Much of the congressional support for care programs for adolescent mothers and their children came from "pro-life" legislators who saw these programs as an alternative to abortions. Certainly the Carter administration's decision to make adolescent pregnancy one of its top domestic priorities can be traced back to their concern about abortion (Vinovskis 1988*a*).

Finally, the role of various interest groups in publicizing the "epidemic" of adolescent pregnancy should not be underestimated. The Alan Guttmacher Institute played a key role in popularizing the phrase "an epidemic of adolescent pregnancy" through its highly influential booklet, *11 Million Teenagers: What Can Be Done about the Epidemic of*

Adolescent Pregnancies in the United States (Alan Guttmacher Institute 1976). Similarly, Eunice Shriver and the Joseph P. Kennedy, Jr., Foundation played an indispensable role in the passage of federally supported care programs for pregnant teenagers.

In other words, while most of the mass media and policymakers incorrectly perceived an unprecedented epidemic of adolescent pregnancy that had appeared in the mid-1970s, they did properly identify a serious social problem that needed assistance. Although the reasons that adolescent pregnancy emerged as one of the top domestic problems are complex and sometimes only indirectly related to the phenomenon itself, the unexpected attention and some resources devoted to this issue were welcomed by many different groups.

Defining the Problem of Adolescent Pregnancy

Although almost everyone today agrees that unintended adolescent pregnancies are a major social problem, there is little consensus on exactly what that problem is or who is responsible for dealing with it. Much of the debate over current policies dealing with adolescent pregnancy is over the definition of the problem and how we should respond to it.

One definition is that sexually active teenagers do not have access to family planning services. While often deploring the recent increases in adolescent sexual activity, proponents of this position assume that there is relatively little that can be done to curb or reduce the current high rates of sexual activity among teenagers. Therefore, the most responsible thing is to provide family planning services to these adolescents in order to prevent any unintended pregnancies.

Providing contraceptive services to teenagers was the primary response of the federal government to adolescent pregnancy in the early 1970s. The passage of the Title X Family Planning Services and Population Research Act of 1970 saw substantial funds directed toward reducing unintended pregnancies among poor women. While the Title X Act did not stress the need for providing contraceptives to unmarried teenagers, in fact nearly a third of its funding was spent in that area (Vinovskis 1988*a*). Reducing adolescent pregnancies through the provision of federally funded contraceptive services became an explicit goal of the Title X Program in 1975 and was reaffirmed strongly in 1978 when the Carter administration proposed shifting family planning funds from poor adult women to adolescents (U.S. Congress, House, Select Committee on Population 1978). Despite the repeated attempts by the Reagan administration to place the Title X Program in a block grant or to reduce its funding, this program continues to be the centerpiece of the federal efforts at dealing with the problem of adolescent pregnancy (Torres and Forrest 1985).

Having failed to alter or reduce the Title X Program, the Reagan administration sought to limit teenagers' access by requiring that parents of patients under eighteen be notified whenever a Title X–funded family planning clinic provided prescription contraceptives to their child. The political battle over this proposed regulation elicited over 120,000 comments and the regulation was finally defeated in the courts (Kenny et al. 1982). While both the administration and its opponents knowingly distorted the effect of the proposed regulations on teenagers, it became an important symbolic issue in regard to the role of parents in dealing with their children (Vinovskis 1988*a*).

Another definition of adolescent pregnancy as a problem is that young mothers and their children are disadvantaged and therefore we should provide care services to help them alleviate the negative consequences of early childbearing. While the proponents of this position are not necessarily opposed to providing family planning services to teenagers, the emphasis is on helping the young mother and her child.

During the 1960s the Children's Bureau sponsored a few demonstration programs designed to help pregnant teenagers and young mothers. Although some of these projects yielded valuable information about the long-term consequences of adolescent pregnancies, they did not have much influence nationally because neither the Johnson nor the Nixon adminstration paid much attention to them (Klerman and Jeckel 1973; Furstenberg, Brooks-Gunn, and Morgan 1987).

Under the leadership of Eunice Shriver and her allies, the federal government gradually expanded its interests in helping school-age mothers. Operating under the incorrect assumption that a large percentage of adolescent pregnancies are intended, Shriver succeeded in convincing the 95th Congress to enact the Title VI Adolescent Health, Services, and Pregnancy Prevention and Care Act of 1978.

Although the Title VI Act was intended both to prevent adolescent pregnancies and to help pregnant teenagers, under the guidance of the first director of the Office of Adolescent Pregnancy Programs, Lulu Mae Nix, it quickly focused almost exclusively on helping pregnant teenagers or young mothers and their infants. The Title VI Program was intended to be a major new social program, with $50 million authorized for FY1979, $65 million FY 1980, and $75 million for FY1981. But the actual appropriations for the program were much more modest—in the range of about $10 million. Although the Title VI Program was placed in a block grant in 1981, a modified version of it survived as a federal demonstration program for providing models to the states on how to deliver care services to pregnant teenagers or to young mothers and their children (Vinovskis 1988a).

A third definition of adolescent pregnancy as a problem is that teenagers are engaging in premarital sexual activity. Proponents of this viewpoint see adolescent sexual activity as the major problem and propose that the local, state, and federal governments should work together with families and churches to reduce early sexual activity. For some of the supporters of this approach, federally funded family planning clinics are seen as a major cause of the recent increases in adolescent sexual activity by seemingly legitimizing early sexual involvement (Kasun 1980).

Although some individuals and groups were upset by the increases in adolescent sexual activity during the 1970s, it was not a major concern of the federal government before the 1980s. In 1981, Senator Jeremiah Denton (R-AL) introduced the Title XX Adolescent Family Life Act that proposed federal funding for experimental programs intended to discourage early sexual activity among teenagers. Dubbed the "Chastity Bill" by its critics, most of the funds for the Title XX Program actually went to support efforts to help pregnant teenagers or to fund social science research.

If the practical effect of the Title XX Program in curtailing early sexual activity is limited, it has had an important symbolic effect on policies dealing with adolescent pregnancies. Despite the concerted outcry against this effort, many individuals and groups now routinely suggest that young teenagers should postpone having sexual intercourse. Furthermore, local, state, and federal officials now also encourage young adolescents to delay early sexual activity—even though most of them privately believe that there is little governments can really do about it.

These three definitions of the problem of adolescent pregnancy have dominated the discussions among policymakers and received the most federal assistance. Although they are not necessarily contradictory in principle, in practice these approaches are often pitted against each other for scarce resources. The debates over their relative merits have also inadvertently limited the exploration of additional issues that warrant further consideration.

For example, there is a growing recognition that the individual who suffers the most in the long term from an adolescent pregnancy is the baby (Furstenberg et al. 1987). Most care programs for pregnant teenagers or young mothers are designed to provide assistance for only one or two years. Although adolescent mothers appear to be more resilient than researchers had initially anticipated, their children are doing much worse as they become adolescents themselves (Furstenberg et al. 1989; but cf. Furstenberg et al. this volume). As a result, future care programs may need to focus more on helping the children of adolescent mothers to escape from the negative consequences of being raised in disadvantaged households.

The other major individual overlooked in our efforts to deal with adolescent pregnancy is the young father. Despite the continued rhetoric about the importance of male involvement, most programs designed to deal with the problems associated with adolescent pregnancy in essence ignore both the responsibilities and the needs of the young father. Indeed, many scholars and policymakers discourage pregnant teenagers from marrying the father as they think this will only compound an already difficult situation (Furstenberg 1988).

There are indications that this neglect of the male role is changing. Increasingly, scholars and policymakers are saying that the young father should be financially accountable for his child whether or not he marries the mother. Although his financial contributions may be very limited initially, they probably will increase substantially over time as his own salary and career progress (Chase-Lansdale and Vinovskis 1987; Furstenberg 1988; Vinovskis and Chase-Lansdale 1988). The current national effort to increase child support payments from absent fathers in general is likely to encourage further developments in this direction, although up to now relatively little attention has been paid to adolescent pregnancies (Chambers 1979; Kahn and Kamerman 1988). Nevertheless, one of the dangers involved in this focus on the financial responsibilities of the father is that it may appear to discourage young fathers from marrying as long as their financial obligations for parenthood are acknowledged and fulfilled.

The other related movement which may have some influence is the new emphasis on the importance of the father in the home (Robinson 1988). Whereas the father was the primary socializer of children in colonial America, today he has been relegated to a minor role in the family (Vinovskis 1986b). Fragmentary research findings suggest that the presence of the father may be an important factor in the satisfactory development of the child and that adolescent mothers who are in a stable marriage are much better off economically (Chase-Lansdale and Vinovskis 1987). While some scholars argue that poor employment opportunities, particularly for black males in the ghettos, is the major reason for the increasing proportion of out-of-wedlock births among teenagers, their evidence is not convincing. Other factors, such as changing cultural attitudes toward marriage and one's sense of responsibility for the consequences of fatherhood, need to be considered as well (Vinovskis 1988*b*). In any case, there is increased interest in redesigning care programs for pregnant teenagers and adolescent mothers and their children in order to help young couples maintain a stable marriage and raise their child.

Conclusion

Young people have always experienced difficulties and tensions as a normal part of growing up. The problems of youth have varied over time in frequency and severity, and the consequences for the individual depend in part on the historical context in which they occurred. But society has not always categorized the problems of young people as the particular difficulties of adolescence. In the past, individual failings were usually seen in more general terms, without teenagers being singled out for special attention or treatment. Adolescent pregnancy, for example, did not emerge as a major social problem for most of the public or policy-makers until the mid-1970s.

Although some teenagers encountered real and serious problems associated with adolescent pregnancy in the past, neither the severity nor the incidence of these difficulties by themselves determined societal reactions. Instead, other factors, such as the changes in birth control technology, the expansion of the rights of young people, the restructuring of the expectations and roles of young women, the increasing costs of welfare dependency, as well as broader social concerns such as the abortion issue help to account for the emergence of the so-called epidemic of adolescent pregnancy as one of the foremost domestic concerns in the late 1970s.

If there is a general consensus today that adolescent pregnancy is harmful to the young couple and their child as well as to society as a whole, there is no agreement on the nature of that problem or the appropriate remedies for it. A glance at the last two decades illustrates how individuals and interest groups differ among themselves in viewing the problem of adolescent pregnancy and how their visions are affected by more general societal trends and changes. Therefore, the debate about adolescent pregnancy is in part an ongoing discourse over who will decide how the problem is defined and who are the individuals and institutions responsible for coping with it.

Since the 1960s the federal government is playing an increasingly active role in dealing with adolescent pregnancies. Several observations can be made about that involvement from a historical perspective. Scholars emphasize the interrelations of different problems of adolescent development and the need to see and treat a troubled teenager as a complex individual, but federal policies and agencies are organized categorically. While the Office of Adolescent Pregnancy Programs (OAPP) focuses on teenage pregnancies, other federal agencies are responsible for dealing with schooling, drug use, juvenile delinquency, and child support enforcement. Although in theory these diverse federal agencies and initiatives are coordinated, in practice they often operate in near-total isolation from each other at both the national and the local levels.

Second, although liberals and conservatives frequently disagree on specific policies, most of them share a strong implicit belief that federal activities are a major factor in creating or alleviating the negative consequences of adolescent pregnancies. They often do not, in both theory and practice, appreciate the influence of larger societal changes and thereby tend to exaggerate the potential effect, positive or negative, of small-scale, federal interventions. Overall shifts in societal attitudes toward sex in general or the role of the mass media in affecting those changes, for example, is slighted compared to the perceived effect of federally funded family planning programs on adolescent sexual behavior. As a result, the debates over any federal initiatives in the area of adolescent pregnancies often seem more like symbolic clashes than realistic proposals to improve the lives of large numbers of teenagers.

Moreover, the nature of the political process in Washington encourages, if not requires, the overstatement of the seriousness of a social problem and the exaggeration of the ability of a limited federal program to solve it. In competing for scarce federal funds, proponents of all particular programs in essence bid against each other through the mass media and congressional hearings about the epidemic proportions of their issues and underestimate the difficulties of coping with them.

In the area of adolescent pregnancy, the unprecedented "epidemic" nature of this crisis was clearly and often deliberately exaggerated in order to garner public and political support. Similarly, earlier statements about 90 percent of the life script of a teenager being determined by an adolescent pregnancy now almost appear as irresponsible claims in light of subsequent research. Such a process of policy-making tends to distort the public's understanding of the complexities of any social problem and encourages us to distrust or discount repeated claims of yet another severe and threatening societal concern that has just been discovered.

Given the frequency with which social problems are identified and overestimated, it is not surprising that policymakers find it tempting and easy to create more small, categorical federal agencies to deal with them—usually knowing full well that not much can or will be really done to solve those problems nationally. This process contributes to the growing cynicism among the public about the efficacy of federal interventions and diverts our attention from the need for more sustained and comprehensive governmental support for disadvantaged individuals and families in our society.

Fourth, some of the participants in the efforts to deal with adolescent pregnancy forget a simple but basic point—it is usually much easier and less expensive, both to the individual and to society, to prevent an unintended pregnancy than to ameliorate the negative consequences of early childbearing. While provisions should be made for helping disadvantaged young couples and their children, most of our efforts should be concentrated on discouraging early sexual activity and encouraging sexually active teenagers to use contraceptives. Although there is a seeming contradiction in telling young teenagers simultaneously to refrain from early sexual activity but to use contraceptives if they do become involved, it is a complex message worth giving and supporting, because once an unintended pregnancy occurs, the remaining options are difficult for many young men and women.

Finally, the federal government and the rest of society should convey a more balanced message to young teenagers about their rights and obligations. On the one hand, adolescents as well as adults are entitled to assistance from their local, state, and federal governments in order to help them develop into good citizens. On the other hand, individuals and families have certain responsibilities for the consequence of their behavior and should be held accountable. Although most of the proponents of increased governmental intervention in the area of adolescent pregnancy focus on what services can and should be provided to teenagers, not enough attention is being given to our expectations about the way those adolescents should behave. For example, if a young man fathers a child, he should share in the financial responsibility for that child for the next eighteen years. Even if his economic contributions are limited initially, a token payment at least establishes unequivocally his responsibility to the mother and the child. At the same time, society has an obligation to assist disadvantaged mothers and young couples in providing decent and stimulating home environments for their children.

There are no easy or simple answers for the problems associated with adolescent pregnancies. A historical approach, however, is useful because it provides us with a broader framework in which to understand the complex interactions between adolescents growing up and the changing social context in which they live. While information about adolescent pregnancies and societal reactions to them in the past should not be used mechanically for guiding current policies, it can sensitize us to the importance of appreciating the effect of larger economic and cultural changes on the lives of teenagers and suggest a broader range of policy options for trying to help our children through their adolescence.

FRANKLIN E. ZIMRING

9   The Jurisprudence of Teenage Pregnancy

In this chapter, any justification there may be for state efforts to have childbearing postponed past the teen years is considered. Then the chapter examines what type of public prevention programs should be pursued. Finally, it deals with the special problems of youth protection that may be produced by policies to discourage teen childbearing.

The chapter thus goes from the abstract to the concrete. Although the opening section may strike some as unnecessarily academic, it may be valuable to define precisely the way we think about justifications for programs and to identify types of public action inconsistent with the rationale behind special state programs.

I believe that our recent experience in reforming the ideas and programs of the juvenile justice system can contribute to a prudent and humane policy toward adolescent pregnancy and parenting. Reform efforts in juvenile justice also provide a broader context in which ideas about teenage pregnancy and its outcomes can be examined and evaluated.

Adolescent Childbearing—A Core Concern

The data presented throughout this book are testament to the special quality of teenage pregnancy and childbearing as a public policy issue.

There have been challenges, however, to the notion that early childbearing is the effective cause of the disadvantages associated with teenage parenting (see Luker 1991).

So a rigorous delineation of what might make teenage parenting a special problem for public law is more than a formal preliminary to the policy analysis of particular kinds of programs. It is important to locate the current concern about teenage childbearing in the modern legal conception of what adolescence is and should mean in the personal development of those who pass through it. We can then use what we regard as the values being protected in worrying about adolescent childbearing as a guide to programs of prevention. Anchoring concerns about teenage childbearing in a specific conception of adolescence helps define the kind of programs that can be justified in the name of this special concern. Moreover, the identification of proper program elements helps us evaluate the consequences of the state's going into the business of discouraging teenage childbearing, consequences, I shall later argue, that do not uniformly operate to the benefit of all young people.

The legal conception of adolescence that I have argued for elsewhere is a period when those not fully adult are engaged in the processes of becoming adult (Zimring 1982). During a period of legal semiautonomy, young persons are progressively given opportunities to make a variety of decisions for themselves, even though it is understood that their relative lack of maturity will lead to a number of errors. This process is justified because trial and error in decision making constitute one necessary part of learning adult competencies in any society where the freedom of choosing the path of one's own life is the hallmark of legal adulthood.

The more complex and multifaceted adult roles become, the longer the learning process to full adult competency, and thus the longer the period of adolescence required for transition into adulthood. This linkage explains the irony that modern adolescents are simultaneously precocious and retarded when compared to earlier cohorts of youth. Much of the rhetoric that accompanied the extension of the franchise to eighteen-year-olds in the early 1970s celebrated the achievement of modern youth, often in contrast with earlier generations. And children today do have more formal education and more exposure to a wider world at earlier ages than the preceding generations.

But there is a contrast between absolute and relative development that characterizes the career of many modern adolescents: the eighteen- or nineteen-year-old of the 1990s typically has achieved more in many spheres of training and development than the eighteen- and nineteen-year-old of the 1920s. But the modern adolescent also typically has further to go to complete the process because of the increasing complexity and variousness of the adult choices that must be made in late twentieth-century American life.

The absolute advantage of the modern adolescent over young people in earlier generations is an argument for earlier exercise of some privileges that depend on minimal competence. However, on a relative basis, intellectual and social development among today's eighteen-year-olds is certainly no closer to the completed process of adult development in the 1990s than was the case in the 1920s or earlier. Young people may have come further, but they also have further to go. The gap that still exists between the equipment for choice possessed by a modern adolescent and what we expect for contemporary adulthood is particularly problematic when we consider those decisions made in adolescence that will have substantial and permanent effect on the life opportunity of young people, decisions such as whether to become a parent.

The juxtaposition of relative and absolute accomplishment is, then, central to the concern about teenage parenthood. In the United States in the 1990s, public concern is expressed not merely about out-of-wedlock pregnancy or pregnancy in the early teens but also about married eighteen- and nineteen-year-old women having babies. This concern has increased, even though the incidence of childbearing in the teen years has not increased recently.

The problem with eighteen-year-old childbearing from this perspective is that early parenthood interrupts the parents' process of development and impinges on the parents' future choices and life chances. Having and keeping a child lock an eighteen-year-old parent into duties and foreclose opportunities. It is this sense of childbearing as arrested development that animates the advertising slogan, "Children having children."

Of course, having a child at any time can lock a parent into commitments of care-giving and will foreclose opportunities for other kinds of development. Having a child before finishing the process of growing up means that the choices between commitments to parenting and to other life opportunities will not be made with the degree of social experience that we associate with adult competence. The decision making that leads to adolescent parenting may be flawed by lack of experience and maturity and is therefore a proper concern of public policy. We want adolescents to accumulate more experience for longer, making decisions with less fateful and permanent consequences in their lives before crossing the threshold of altruistic permanent commitment.

In this account, the central problem of premature commitments to parenting relates to the quality of decision making. Persons who become parents give up other opportunities as a consequence at whatever stage in their social development the decision is made. The problem of teenage parenting is that the decision to forgo other opportunities is not made with the same wideness of worldview and the same experience in making decisions that are the hallmark of adulthood in democratic society.

There are, of course, some persons who make decisions in the same way at age eighteen that they would at age twenty-five or thirty. This may well be as true of some sixteen-year-olds. But for most modern adolescents, the world widens dramatically during the years of secondary school and just beyond. In an ideology of adolescence that places great emphasis on mobility and choice, there is great personal cost in making binding choices earlier than when the range of choice available is well known.

This broad objection to adolescent parenting can be contrasted with two narrower sets of concerns that focus on the association between teen parenting and manifest pathology. One concern about "children having children" is that an interruption in the maturing process of the teenage parent will lead to unfortunate near-term consequences. Thus, we hear that those who become parents at young ages will interrupt their educations and forgo economic opportunities as a consequence of childbearing.

Two points can be made about this. First, becoming a parent carries opportunity costs throughout the life cycle. Adult decisions to bear and raise children also frequently lead to sacrifice in educational and economic opportunities for parents. A measure of respect is frequently paid to adult citizens who choose to make the sacrifices associated with becoming parents. Why, then, our paternalistic hostility to the sacrifices of teenage childbearing? The emphasis on the quality of decision making involved in becoming a parent provides an answer. The social plaint about adolescent decisions to forgo other opportunities in order to become parents is "You don't know what you're missing."

A second point is made that there are some lost opportunities associated with premature childbearing that do not occur in later periods. Even if the young mother manages to finish school and find a desirable job, the process of deciding to become a parent will lack the resonance of maturity. Having come to parenthood too early, she will find that the path to making the decision will not contain the experienced-based reflection that itself then becomes one of the positive aspects of later parenthood. In this view, immaturity can render the decision to bear children as lacking truly informed consent.

An even narrower set of concerns about adolescent childbearing involves a high incidence of particular identified pathologies such as low birth weight, impaired maternal and child health, welfare dependency, illegitimacy, near-term divorce, and the like. These special problems exacerbate adolescent pregnancy far too often, and additional resources should be invested in programs aimed at postponing parenthood beyond the adolescent years on account of these related pathologies (Hamburg and Dixon, this volume).

But if this litany of pathologies is the heart of the matter, then a special concern with adolescent pregnancy is both overinclusive and underinclusive. It is over-inclusive because some adolescent childbearing will avoid serious pathology. This is particularly the case when public resources are invested to support childbearing. And a targeted concern on adolescent pregnancy is also underinclusive in that the majority of children from divorced and welfare-dependent families are not the direct result of teenage childbearing. A focused concern on pathological outcome would seem to be as much directed at support for parenting by young persons as for postponing parenting. It would also miss some aspects of adolescent development worth notice.

Cause for Concern?

There is ample room on the basis of currently available data to disagree about the importance of early childbearing as an independent problem meriting public intervention. Many of the handicaps associated with early child rearing are not necessarily caused by pregnancy and parenting (Luker 1991). And many of the educational and experiential options we could wish for middle and late adolescents would not be widely available to young mothers in any event because of their limited economic means and educational background. In this sense, the theory of adolescence that animates a general objection to early childbearing can be seen as restrictively middle-class.

Yet the aspirations that most urban households of all classes have for their children are also rather middle-class, and there are few enclaves in late twentieth-century America where an eighteen-year-old's pregnancy is regarded as good news by parents and peers. While becoming a parent in the late teen years can be something less than a disaster (Furstenberg et al. 1987), a public preference to keep the teen years occupied with the adolescent's personal development can be justified. Nobody yet argues that teenage childbearing facilitates choice and mobility. The fact that early childbearing is by no means the only restriction on development faced by adolescents at risk requires broader programs than just pregnancy prevention. But social comfort with other people's children being locked into permanent roles while our own children preserve middle-class options seems a far from benign double standard.

That the costs of teen parenting may have been overestimated becomes an argument against public investment in prevention only if such prevention programs hurt young people. This highlights the important relationship between the justification for public programs in this area and the content and effects of the programs. My own conclusion is that as long as a public program pays proper regard to the interests of the kids it is trying to protect, a policy to encourage postponing childbearing beyond the teen years can be justified.

Implications for Program Strategy

The decision to have children at any age carries significant opportunity costs. In America the opportunity costs of adolescent childbearing are seen to be higher than for childbearing in later years. But whether or not the burdens encountered by an adolescent parent are greater, there is a separate justification for special public concern about adolescent parenting because adolescents lack the life experiences that would prepare them for making so fateful a choice in an authentically adult way. Adolescent parents do not know what they would be missing.

If this concern functions as the justification for special state programs, I argue that the programs designed to respond to this problem should be: (1) general in scope rather than simply targeting the earlier years of adolescence; (2) preventive rather than just ameliorative; (3) paternalistic in preferring postponed parenthood; and (4) protective of the adolescent at risk rather than punitive or neutral in approach.

Generality

A concern with the quality of decision making about childbearing can support programs that encompass the full range of adolescent development rather than the earlier adolescent years that are of particularly high biological and economic risk. No matter what one's special orientation, early adolescence presents particularly high risks for pregnancy and parenting. The concern for "children having children" is most acute when those children are thirteen-, fourteen-, and fifteen-year-olds, still early in the secondary education process, still not physically mature, and great distances away from the experiential base that should be the background for decisions about marriage and childbearing. Any program especially concerned with adolescent pregnancy should make young adolescents a special priority.

But a concern about the proper experiential background for decisions about having a child need not be restricted to younger adolescents. Publicly supported programs that are based on the concerns outlined earlier can and should target older adolescents as well as younger ones and express concern about decisions made by high school graduates as well as younger adolescents. In this sense, adolescents who are not obviously regarded as still "children" should be the object of concern about childbearing decisions even if they are already acquiring job experience, voting in national elections, and further along the way to authentic adulthood than the younger teens (Zimring 1982).

Prevention

Another feature of the public programs that can be justified on this ground is that they are concerned with prevention as well as the amelioration of the problems associated with adolescent pregnancy and childbearing. If only the lack of prenatal care would justify special concerns for adolescent pregnancy, why not concentrate public funding on providing prenatal care instead of attempting to reduce the incidence of pregnancy? Similarly, if the limited economic opportunity associated with teenage parenting was the major concern, why not just invest public funds to provide counseling and other supportive services?

Concern for premature judgment suggests the investment of resources to prevent pregnancy, not just to support teen pregnancy and parenting. This is especially true for younger adolescents, but also justified for those of our children who are well launched in college and on the development of a variety of experiences in travel, education, and dating.

Paternalism

The special justification for postponing adolescent child rearing permits a degree of paternalism in the administration of prevention programs, although there are important practical and principled limits to the degree of paternalism that should be allowed. The limited paternalism I support is one of a state program that can persist in preferring the postponement of childbearing among adolescents even if the adolescents disagree. If the problematic nature of adolescent judgment about childbearing is the justification for a special program, it would be inconsistent to simultaneously premise a special program on notions of immaturity of judgment and to exempt all adolescents who wish to have children from a public judgment that family responsibility should be deferred.

But it is only in this special case that notions of adolescent immaturity provide an automatic basis for substituting public judgments for personal preferences. Once pregnancy is an accomplished fact, any presumption that the state knows best should probably be inoperative. The limited case paternalism I support is limited to preferring that children do not get pregnant.

Why not let notions of adolescent immaturity license more forceful varieties of state intervention? Let me defer this issue briefly while finishing the list of themes implied by the central concern outlined in the first section.

Protection

My final implied dimension of public programs is the most important. State initiatives in this field should protect the individual adolescent at risk rather than be punitive or neutral with respect to her immediate welfare interests. If the reason we worry about adolescents becoming parents is the risk to their welfare as adults then the welfare of the individual adolescent should remain central in a special program. Public programs designed merely to reduce welfare rolls or infant mortality or divorce rates should not be targeted especially at adolescents. The special concern of adolescent childbearing is adolescent welfare, and the obligation that the state authority assumes in taking special power over the lives of adolescents on this account is to do so with their welfare as a central policy goal.

With this point about youth welfare in mind, we can return to the real-world context of limited paternalism. What prevents society from implementing paternalistic programs aimed at adolescents at risk for childbearing that are both compulsory and therapeutic? The objection to this combination of coercive state programs as the means and youth welfare as the end is a practical one. Three-quarters of a century of juvenile court reform efforts have been founded on the futility of coercing cures among the young. More specifically, the adolescent at risk of pregnancy has long been considered what the law calls a "status offender" and was made the subject of compulsory public programs that were celebrated failures in protecting the adolescent and the larger community (Zimring 1982). There is in this history no evidence available that compulsory programs that greatly restrict the liberty of adolescents at risk achieve benefits worth their substantial costs.

The history of efforts to coercively cure status offenders suggests that the burden of persuasion should be substantial on those who would return to government efforts in that direction. But history also suggests that new emphasis on a peril to adolescent development is frequently accompanied by new bursts of faith in coercive intervention. Changing the problem label seems to reinvigorate enthusiasm for policies of coercion.

Broad powers were delegated to the juvenile courts to deal with large categories of adolescents at risk. Institutions were built and staffed, programs were funded and widely praised on the assumption that paternalistic and coercive programs could rescue adolescents from the danger of living criminal, immoral, and dissolute lives.

The best historical evidence demonstrates that coercive intervention programs never worked (Schlossman 1977). The contemporary effort to rethink government's role in dealing with status offenders emphasizes reduction in forced intervention while attempting to minimize the real dangers that status offenders face in unregulated environments with voluntary programs and limited crisis intervention.

The consensus that supports this direction of reform for status offender programs is all the more remarkable because of society's reluctance to accept the limited capacity of the state to help adolescents at risk. A sense of limit conflicts with the persistent American optimism that only the right set of programs need be identified for problems to be solved.

Thus, there is more than a small danger that the relabeling of problems and the programs designed to respond to them can lead to a repetition of the mistakes that characterized earlier adventures with status offenders. With each new threat to adolescent well-being—be it an epidemic of teenage pregnancy, the threat of crack cocaine, or the specter of AIDS—impulses to intervene run high. Often, the institutional memory of program failures does not carry over to the new institutions participating in policy discussion and in the arena of legislative change. For this reason, one hazard in public policy toward adolescents in the United States is that it is merely old wine in new bottles.

The Perils of Prevention

Those who design and execute criminal laws have a much easier task than the practitioners of juvenile justice in one important respect. The goal of criminal law is to stigmatize particular forms of proscribed behavior as well as the persons who engage in that behavior. To cast both the act and the actor in the same negative light is often possible. But the law gives those who practice juvenile justice an unattainable goal, the objective of stigmatizing behaviors without stigmatizing those young persons who engage in them. The goal is unattainable because negative social judgments about particular behaviors inevitably spill over to become social evaluations of the persons who engage in those behaviors.

This social fact has placed a contradiction at the heart of the operation of twentieth-century juvenile justice: What the formal law demands— stigma-free treatment of the alleged delinquent—cannot be achieved when the system simultaneously wishes to attach stigma to delinquent behavior. Even in an age that has witnessed a so-called Teflon presidency, social judgments about delinquent behavior inevitably rub off on those who engage in the behavior.

The same conflict can be seen at the center of programs that seek to reduce rates of adolescent pregnancy yet ameliorate the difficult life settings of adolescents who are involved in the process. Effective prevention programs will stigmatize teen childbearing. That negative social judgment puts pregnant and childbearing adolescents at greater risk. One consequence of this is that a major secondary goal of preventive programs in this area should be the correction of the negative effects that are by-products of a primary prevention thrust.

Do successful prevention programs really stigmatize adolescent parenting? Of course. Any program that seeks to redirect voluntary adolescent behavior is an exercise in marketing. With respect to adolescent parenting, the marketing task is to focus attention on the negative aspects of pregnancy, childbearing, and child rearing. Some analogues in our recent experience are public and private campaigns to dissuade teenagers from cigarette smoking and, more recently, using drugs. The antismoking campaign research found that the most successful appeals to an adolescent audience involved short-term rather than long-term effects and emphasized the dumbness of smoking. The marketing task is to convince young persons that those of their peers who smoke should not be emulated. The mechanism is stigma.

So, one necessary element of discouraging teenage parenting is stigma. But negative messages about adolescent pregnancy and child rearing inevitably spill over into negative judgments about pregnant and parenting teens. Programs that effectively dissuade young persons at risk of becoming parents do so at the price of further lowering the social standing of those who are pregnant and parents.

One case study in the manifest and latent effect of stigma involves teenage marriage. If the last four decades of American demographic experience were to become a Perry Mason adventure, it could be titled

"The Case of the Disappearing Bridegroom." As figure 9.1 shows, the number of girls, aged fifteen to nineteen, who are currently married has declined in each census year since mid-century and now stands at miniscule levels (U.S. Bureau of the Census 1953; Hayes 1987). Behaviorally, teenage marriage is social deviance in the late 1980s, which seems to have reduced the birthrate among teenage girls thus deferring childbearing to later years for many young women (see, e.g., Weeks 1976).

But as marriage rates decline, a larger proportion of those pregnancies that do occur during the teen years will occur outside of marriage. In this sense, an increase in the proportion of all live births among teenage girls that are illegitimate is evidence that policies that stigmatize teenage marriages are working, but working at a substantial cost to a group of young women who are pregnant, unmarried, and the object of social stigma.

Consider, for example, the social environment in which an eighteen-year-old male high school senior makes a decision in the 1990s about how to respond to the fact that his seventeen-year-old girlfriend is pregnant. Demographic statistics suggest that the young man bent on "doing the right thing" in the 1950s frequently reached different decisions than he reaches in the 1990s. And one important reason for this is that the social status of marrying at eighteen in order to raise a child has declined precipitously. However difficult in other respects, one of the nice things about "doing the right thing" is the positive judgment one obtains from one's social group after embarking on that course of action. That kind of positive reinforcement for eighteen-year-old males marrying seems to have disappeared from adult society and from most adolescent peer cultures in the United States.

The simple point is this: The war on adolescent pregnancy necessarily inflicts casualties, and today these casualties are pregnant and childbearing adolescents. These teenage girls were always at the highest risk of suffering the bad outcomes that come with early parenting. One negative consequence of stigma-based programs is increased difficulties suffered by those most at risk of negative social consequences from teenage pregnancy. What to do?

There is a direct contradiction between the negative effects of stigma-based prevention programs and any sentiment that initiatives in this field should be protective of the individual adolescent at risk. One way to cope with this kind of conflict is to deny the protective obligation of state policy. Thus, in dealing with delinquents, some contemporary observers now use the blameworthiness of individual delinquents to deny any

FIGURE 9.1

Percent of Women, 15–19, Who Have Ever Been Married, by Race and Census Year

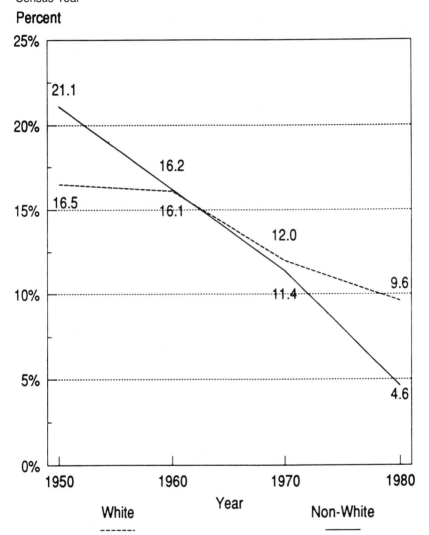

Data for 1950 are from U.S. Bureau of the Census (1953); data for 1960, 1970, and 1980 are from Hayes (1987).

obligation to take their interests into account in the juvenile justice process. Can a parallel argument be constructed for disowning those who are dumb enough to get pregnant or to stay pregnant? I hope not, but blaming the victim is tempting in social policy toward adolescents at risk.

Instead, a balanced social agenda requires programs to ameliorate the risks experienced by girls who experience pregnancy in adolescence. This obligation should be a reason to avoid inflicting gratuitous stigma in programs (i.e., by excluding adolescent mothers from educational programs). The obligation to protect provides another reason to justify programs for those males and females who choose adolescent parenting as the lesser evil.

But is it not inconsistent to support both programs that seek to prevent adolescent parenting and programs that seek to support young persons who have children? The answer is, no. As long as youth welfare is the goal of pregnancy prevention programs, the same reasons that underlie committing resources to prevention programs counsel us to help those of our older children who now have children themselves. If we value the developmental options of young people, we should seek public policies that foster the development of pregnant as well as non-pregnant young women.

The true inconsistency is pursuing youth welfare only to the water's edge, by using the needs of young persons as a justification for prevention programs but ignoring those needs when pregnancy and childbirth occur. Both support of adolescent parenting and steps toward prevention are necessary elements of an evenhanded policy that addresses the central social harm of premature parenting.

EVELYN Z. BRODKIN

10 Teen Pregnancy and the Dilemmas of Social Policymaking

In a perfectly ordered policy world, one might imagine that social conditions would receive attention in proportion to their scope and seriousness. In the real world, this relationship is highly problematic and has been subject to serious analytic scrutiny by students of social policymaking.[1] A major theme of this scholarship is that social policies are only partially responsive to social conditions. Policies also are responsive to the politics of the policymaking process, which presents strategic dilemmas to policy advocates as they move through stages of the process from agenda-setting to coalition-building to implementation. The prospects and hazards of fashioning policy responses to teen pregnancy and childbearing can be better understood if these dilemmas and their implications are clarified.

This chapter draws on the valuable contributions to this volume by Professors Vinovskis and Zimring to illuminate ways in which policymaking for teen pregnancy has been shaped not only by substantive considerations, but also by strategic dilemmas of the policymaking process. Two broad propositions presented and briefly discussed below provide a schematic for clarifying these dilemmas and considering their policy implications.

Among other things, this approach draws attention to the fact that the "problem" of teen pregnancy, like other social concerns, is subject to multiple definitions, each having different political and policy implications. The terms "teen pregnancy," "adolescent childbearing," and "teenage parenthood" each in some way labels or presupposes the parameters of the problem it seeks to describe—whether it is one of teenagers or adolescents, pregnancy or childbearing, childbearing or parenting. These terms do not directly raise issues that some argue more accurately define "the problem," for example, social stigma, poverty, racism, or sexism. In lieu of a suitably generic term, I use the conventional terms employed in the general literature but, in the course of discussion, take note of the divergent assumptions embedded in those terms.

The Agenda-setting Dilemma

Proposition: Problem definitions that draw attention to an issue enhance its prospects of winning a place on a crowded policy agenda but create difficulties for policy formulation by mobilizing diverse groups with competing interests.[2]

E. E. Schattschneider (1960) once succinctly summarized politics as "the mobilization of bias." One dictum that may be derived from his rich analysis is that the attention and active engagement of potential supporters must be mobilized if a social issue is to move successfully from the private to the public sphere and through the policymaking process. Stated differently, the advancement of a social issue onto the policy agenda is enhanced by maximizing attention and political mobilization.[3] However, the mobilization of political attention and the activation of support are difficult to achieve and even harder to sustain. This is particularly true in social politics, in part because potential policy beneficiaries tend to be those with the least political power and fewest social or economic resources.[4]

The literature on agenda setting suggests three related elements— only one of which is endogenous to the issue itself—that contribute to the mobilization of attention and support in a crowded policy environment. They are: (1) the way an issue is defined (Cobb and Elder 1975; Nelson 1984; Hilgartner and Bosk 1988; Stone 1989); (2) the interests of relevant institutions or the people who run them (Walker 1977; Kingdon 1984; Nelson 1984); and (3) the availability of a "policy window" (Kingdon 1984).

Issue Definition

In some cases, the proximate cause propelling an issue to agenda status may be fairly evident. Cobb and Elder (1975) refer to "triggering events" that dramatically bring an issue to public consciousness. These events include natural catastrophes such as floods or earthquakes and man-made crises such as acts of war, assassinations, or coups d'etat. Unambiguous triggering events like these rarely, if ever, explain the origins of social issues. More often, conditions that constitute potential social issues develop gradually or fester chronically, as in the case of homelessness, hunger, child abuse, or poverty. Although these may be defined as crises, as in the "crisis of teen pregnancy," the crisis designation can be better understood as a political construct that responds to strategic imperatives of agenda setting than as a description accurately reflecting the dramatic onset of a social problem.

For example, examining teen pregnancy in historical perspective, Vinovskis demonstrates that the rising rhetoric of the teen pregnancy crisis was not accompanied by a dramatic escalation in the incidence of teen pregnancy or childbirth. In fact, the issue emerged on the policy agenda at the same time that the scope of the purported problem appeared to diminish. This is anomalous if one assumes that social conditions drive agenda setting. But what if one assumes instead that political and institutional factors drive agenda setting? In that case, one would look elsewhere to understand why and how the issue arose.

The literature on agenda setting suggests that issues are most likely to achieve agenda status if they are defined in relatively nontechnical terms and as having relatively broad social significance, wide-ranging effects, and immediate consequences (Cobb and Elder 1975). It is also advantageous if they are accompanied by proposed remedies that do not require a major departure from existing practice (ibid.). These characteristics can be identified readily in definitions of the teen pregnancy crisis, although the definitions vary considerably.

From this perspective, the contradiction Vinovskis demonstrates between declining teen childbirth and the declaration of a public crisis of teen pregnancy should not be altogether surprising. If the crisis designation seems anomalous in the context of objective social "facts," it would appear quite congruent with the strategic imperative of agenda setting, that is, the need to attract public attention to an issue through dramatic, even overstated, presentation of a problem (Hilgartner and Bosk 1988).

The designation of a crisis itself suggests the immediacy and urgency of the problem and implies that its effects will widen if unattended.

Proclamation of crisis often marks the first sally of a policy debate, as, for example, in the welfare crisis, environmental crisis, fiscal crisis, urban crisis, and so forth. The "crisis-of-the-month club" may have a floating membership, but it is one with a common strategic interest in attention getting.[5] To more fully understand the appearance of crises in social policy discourse, it is important to consider the interests and resources of relevant institutional actors.

Institutional Interests

While dramatization of an issue may be a necessary condition for winning a place on the policy agenda, it is not generally a sufficient one. An issue's prospects also are enhanced by the active interest of resource-rich institutional and political actors. Institutions—such as government agencies, professional groups, or service providers—often have a stake in issues that may bring them expanded budgets and authority or protect their professional turf. Among their agenda-setting resources, these institutions tend to have visibility, professional standing, and credibility. At times, an emergent social issue may offer a vehicle that enables institutions to promote an earlier set of interests. For example, Nelson (1984) emphasizes the importance to the Children's Bureau of capturing the child abuse issue in the 1960s as a means of maintaining the bureau's dwindling public health role and, in effect, maintaining the agency's own health.

In the case of teen pregnancy, Vinovskis hints at the role played by institutional actors using the teen pregnancy issue to pursue related interests. In particular, he points to the Guttmacher Institute, which popularized the notion of a teen pregnancy "epidemic," and to the Shriver and Kennedy Foundation, as advancing their prior family planning interests through this issue. Equally intriguing, Vinovskis suggests that the teen pregnancy issue may have partly developed as a proxy engagement in the ongoing battle over abortion. He contends that the Carter administration's choice of adolescent pregnancy as a major domestic priority stemmed from the Department of Health and Human Services' search for an alternative path around the politically charged abortion controversy.

Policy Windows

Kingdon uses the term "policy window" to describe an opportunity for advancing an issue, a window that opens infrequently and does not remain open for long (Kingdon 1984). This element of the policy environment is closely related to the definitional and institutional elements outlined above. A policy window may open because an issue has been defined in a way that captures media and public attention, as in various "crises." It also may open in response to the efforts of institutional and political entrepreneurs who have a strong interest in an issue and the resources to pursue it.

The fundamental interest of politicians and executives in credit-claiming gives them an incentive to attempt to exploit open policy windows or seek to open them.[6] Again, the chapter by Vinovskis is suggestive in this regard, especially with respect to the secretary of Health and Human Services and his interest in diverting attention from the abortion issue. It should be noted that the self-interest of issue entrepreneurs is often coupled with substantive, philosophical, or other complementary interest in the matter. However, the latter types of interest may not alone be sufficient to induce entrepreneurial activity.

The Coalition Formation Dilemma

Proposition: Policy proposals that oversimplify problems, overstate solutions, and mask competing objectives may help promote coalition-building necessary to advance policies through the legislative process; but such policies, when enacted, create potential implementation difficulties, public dissatisfaction and even political backlash.

If the central imperative of agenda setting is to expand and intensify active interest in a social policy issue, the strategic responses to that imperative create problems for the next stage of the policy process. Social issues defined dramatically to provoke attention and to serve the interests of various institutional actors may be poorly defined to meet the coalition-building requirements of legislative or agency policymaking. Coalition building is enhanced by limiting conflict, bridging opposing interests, and minimizing political and fiscal costs. But once the scope of conflict is expanded in the agenda-setting process, how can it be limited in the legislative process? Once institutions have defined issues according to their own interests, how can competing interests be reconciled? Once issues have been defined as critical and broad in scope, how can the costs of addressing them be minimized?

Responses . . .

One strategic response to these questions is to define a social policy issue in terms that are more consensual than conflictual, more technical than manifestly political. Defining a condition as an illness or pathology—that is, "medicalizing" a condition—promotes consensus by depoliticizing it, lends credibility to the notion that "experts" can "cure" it, and helps to limit "legitimate" participation to those conversant with the language of experts. For example, as Nelson (1984) convincingly demonstrates in her analysis of the child abuse issue, labeling abuse as a medical syndrome helped policymakers circumvent contentious issues concerning the criminality of abusers, the role of the state in family life, and possible social causes of abuse. According to Nelson (1984), the identification of a "battered-child syndrome," first reported in medical journals, helped to "diffuse anxiety and promote consensus through the choice of a nonthreatening label" (59). Medicalization of the issue also enabled a coalition of institutional interests including the Children's Bureau, physicians, and researchers to fashion remedies that would be consistent with their own practices and institutional interests (Nelson 1984). As a fringe benefit, medicalization of a problem makes it appear susceptible to expert treatment and, by implication, subject to remedy within normal modes of practice.

Despite its strategic advantages, the drawbacks to the medicalization of social issues are impressive. As Arthur Kohrman (1988) has pointed out, applying a medical model to a social problem may lead to incorrect diagnosis of causation and misdirected remedies. For example, Kohrman makes a crucial distinction between diagnosing the cause of behaviors leading to teen pregnancy as "depression" versus "hopelessness." Depression, he explains, defines a clinical condition that produces dysfunctional behaviors and is subject to treatment at an individual level. In contrast, hopelessness defines a response to structural conditions, such as poverty or discrimination, that indicate a social rather than an individual pathology and require a social solution.

Apparently dysfunctional behaviors, when viewed as responses to adverse structural conditions, may be reinterpreted as functional in the sense that they provide a means of coping with an environment that offers few, if any, of the positive options routinely available to individuals with more social advantages. Teenage pregnancy may constitute an affirmative act for some poor young women who see few opportunities for the types of personal development commonly available to nonpoor women (Dash 1989; Hamburg and Dixon this volume). If Kohrman's distinction between depression and hopelessness is correct, then policies that adopt a medicalized definition of the phenomenon will misdirect attention to changing the behavior of poor young women rather than attacking their poverty.

A second strategic response to the coalition-building imperative is to overstate the problem while understating the difficulties of addressing it in a meaningful way. This takes into account the general interest of politicians in credit-claiming, which leads them to favor issues that appear to be "high salience, low cost" (Price 1978). From this perspective, an issue's prospects of advancing through the policy process are enhanced if it can be defined as significant but framed in sufficiently consensual terms to minimize political opposition and in sufficiently narrow terms to minimize fiscal costs.[7]

. . . *And Consequences*

One consequence of "high salience, low cost" coalition-building strategies is that apparent policy achievements may turn out to be more symbolic than real. For one thing, policymakers may appear to be addressing a problem but fail to provide adequate financial resources. For example, Vinovskis's brief history of the Title X Family Planning and Population Research Act suggests that politicians were able to claim credit for policymaking without ever appropriating the funding authorized by the act.

For another thing, policies responding to the coalition-building imperative often contain ambiguous or contradictory objectives, essentially referring to implementing agencies critical elements of what policy-in-practice will be (Brodkin 1990). For example, Vinovskis points to the mixed set of family planning and service objectives contained in Title X. Upon implementation, he asserts, these multiple objectives were largely reduced to dissemination of contraceptives, an objective that reflected the institutional interests of policy implementers.

Zimring's approach to the teen pregnancy issue offers an interesting and complex response to the strategic dilemmas described here. In presenting a normative rationale for public policies to prevent teen pregnancy, he attempts to derive the strategic advantages of "medicalizing" the issue while minimizing its disadvantages. He proposes to define adolescent childbearing as a problem of adolescent development. Like the battered-child syndrome in the child abuse example, Zimring's "arrested development syndrome" avoids issues of morality and builds on jurisprudential precedents that legitimate a protective state role in caring for adolescents. It also largely sidesteps the matter of possible social causes of teen pregnancy and implies that the problem, at least partially, can be "treated" at the individual level.[8]

On the other hand, Zimring explicitly eschews victim blaming and recalls the sorry history of legal approaches to pregnant teens that labeled them "status offenders" (if they were not married) and justified coercive and stigmatizing interventions. He is hopeful that reformist approaches to juvenile justice generally will encourage more balanced responses to adolescent pregnancy now. But, he wisely cautions, "there is more than a small danger that the relabeling of problems and the programs designed to respond to them can lead to a repetition of the mistakes that characterized earlier adventures with status offenders" (Zimring this volume).

There also remains the danger that, by formulating the issue of teen pregnancy as one of protecting adolescent development, a broad consensus may be achieved, but only by masking fundamental disagreement about whether the problem is primarily one of individual dysfunction or, rather, one emerging from structural inequalities in society and the economy. Although individual and structural issues need not be viewed as strictly dichotomous, coalition formation strategies that fail to resolve such fundamental matters are likely to produce policies of dubious value in addressing social problems to which they can only partially respond.

The ultimate ambiguity of policy-in-practice after a winning coalition has been forged and political credit has been claimed constitutes a major dilemma for social policymaking. Ambiguous policies or policies with multiple and conflicting objectives effectively leave the task of resolving ambiguities and conflicts to the discretion of those responsible for policy implementation. In effect, policy choices avoided in the course of the legislative policymaking process are delegated down the policy chain to be made, often implicitly, by those implementing policy at the state, local, or street level (Brodkin 1990). Perhaps paradoxically, both the strength and the weakness of Zimring's approach derives from its reliance on the exercise of professional judgment by policy implementers. Policies that delegate discretion to social welfare providers may, in some cases, be superior to those that attempt to specify rules and apply them uniformly to categories of individuals. But ambiguous policies run the risk that the policy "balance" produced at the point of delivery may not be compatible with the policy vision of its authors.

Appreciation of this dilemma makes one skeptical of the outcome of the "balanced" policy approach that Zimring advocates. Whatever its intrinsic merits, a balanced policy that neither stigmatizes nor glorifies, that offers support but within the parameters of limited paternalism, is likely to have more strategic utility for coalition building than for producing specific policy activities at the point of implementation. The implications of the coalition-building dilemma for this and other proposals merit careful consideration.

Further Reflections on Policymaking for Teen Pregnancy

The strategic imperatives of social policymaking present difficult dilemmas for those who seek to address various aspects of the teen pregnancy problem. First, constructions of "the problem" that advance the issue onto the policy agenda—in particular, those that intimate a crisis or epidemic—may mobilize groups with competing views of and interests in the matter that are difficult to reconcile at the policymaking stage. Then, too, constructions of policy solutions that enable coalitions to form around specific proposals and potentially permit political credit-claiming at low cost may produce policies containing ambiguous or contradictory objectives and resources insufficient to deal meaningfully with problems. Third, as Vinovskis suggests, strategies used to overcome indifference to social problems and political stalemate, by overstating problems and understating the resources needed to address them, may lead to disappointment and backlash. Ironically, this may diminish prospects for dealing with the problem in the future.

This does not mean that no response is better than an imperfect response. To contend that the dilemmas of social policymaking logically constitute an argument in behalf of reprivatizing social problems too conveniently overlooks the great human and political costs of leaving these problems unattended. The more productive alternative is to carefully consider policy issues in light of the strategic dilemmas outlined in this chapter both when conceptualizing social problems and when proposing policy solutions. Greater understanding of the dilemmas of social policymaking may improve chances to avoid some of the worst pitfalls and seize some of the best opportunities.

NOTES

1. A central thrust of research on agenda setting and social policymaking is to investigate the factors, both endogenous and exogenous to the issues themselves, that effect issue identification and recognition as well as policy adoption. See, for example, Brodkin (1990), Cobb and Elder (1975), Crenson (1971), Heclo (1978), Hilgartner and Bosk (1988), Kingdon (1984), Nelson (1984), Stone (1989), Walker (1977). The notion of strategic dilemmas I develop here is meant to concentrate analytic attention on those political and institutional factors that influence the content and progress of the policy process independent of the motives or intent of policy participants. It does not assume that policy

advocates are cynically playing games to advance their own positions, although at times they may be.

2. The concept of agendas has been variously defined to distinguish between a "systemic agenda" that includes issues generally recognized to be matters for public concern and a "governmental, action, or policy agenda" that includes issues under active consideration by a legislature or policy agency (Cobb and Elder 1975; Nelson 1984).

3. Schattschneider (1960) explains that it is the losing side in any conflict that has a strategic interest in expanding the scope of conflict to enlarge its support. For those benefiting disproportionately from the status quo, it is preferable to narrow the scope of conflict. Under these circumstances, it generally follows that policymaking on behalf of the socially disadvantaged would benefit from expanded mobilization. In contrast, the privatization of social problems would favor the prevailing distribution of social and economic power. For an elaboration of these points, see, in addition to Schattschneider, Crenson (1971), Gamson (1975), and Starr and Immergut (1987).

4. For varying perspectives on the obstacles posed by "issue-attention cycles," "collective action problems," and inequality, see Downs (1972), Gamson (1975), Olson (1965), and Pateman (1970).

5. A disjuncture between crisis rhetoric and reality is not unusual. For example, public proclamations of a welfare crisis reached a crescendo in the early 1970s, just as the growth in welfare caseloads had leveled off (Rein and Heclo 1973). For examples of crisis formation in other areas, including environmental policy, urban policy and foreign policy, respectively, see Brodkin and Shaikh (1986), Piven (1974), and Lowi (1967).

6. For example, Nelson notes that when Walter Mondale was named chair of the Senate Subcommittee on Children and Youth, he looked for an issue that he could effectively pursue in his new committee role and that might eventually further his presidential ambitions (Nelson 1984). Illuminating assessments of entrepreneurship by politicians and agency executives also can be found in Heclo (1978), Kingdon (1984), Lynn (1986), and Price (1978).

7. Nelson (1984) credits the speed with which the issue of child abuse gathered support and produced legislation to precisely these issue characteristics. However, she also blames those issue characteristics for contributing to an inadequate policy response—one that failed to resolve conflicting interpretations of the problem or provide sufficient institutional and financial resources to address it.

8. Zimring's reference to the opportunity costs of early childbearing appears to refer to the opportunities young people lose or trade off when they become parents. However, it is precisely the lack of opportunity for poor youths (other than the opportunity to have a child) that Kohrman, Furstenberg, and others emphasize. These contrasting perspectives have significantly different policy implications—the first suggesting interventions aimed at individual behaviors, the second suggesting interventions aimed at the social and economic structure of opportunity.

KYU-TAIK SUNG

11 Teenage Pregnancy and Premarital Childbirth in Korea: Issues and Concerns

Attitudes toward Out-of-Wedlock Pregnancy and Childbirth

The social and health care services available to a social group depend very much on the values prevalent in the larger society of which it is a part. In spite of the national resources that Korea has accumulated—a large pool of trained personnel and increasing wealth—the nation has not yet developed viable and effective human service programs for dealing with the subgroup of young, high-risk women who become unmarried mothers.

The public attitude in Korea toward unmarried mothers and pregnant teenagers remains very negative. Koreans are reluctant to accept and recognize sexual relations among young people outside marriage, not to mention the troublesome consequences thereof. The people of Korea have a long tradition of family care and communal support, and they are generally humane, sympathetic, and helpful to each other. However, they have not demonstrated the same cultural traits in dealing with unmarried mothers and pregnant teenagers. The negative attitude is dying hard.

Positive attitudes toward teenage pregnancies are not something that can be instituted by human service professionals alone. Change must take place in the minds and behaviors of all members of society. More positive attitudes toward unmarried pregnant young women must be promoted in the general public. If policies and programs emanated from a more positive perspective on teenage mothers and unmarried mothers, more resources would be used to provide more effective services, and the quality and quantity of the services would reflect that positive perspective.

The following story will give some idea of general attitudes in Korea about unmarried pregnancy and the difficult situation in which most unmarried young mothers find themselves.[1]

A sixteen-year-old schoolgirl in Seoul became pregnant but had little understanding of what was happening to her. (Sex education is still limited in Korea.) When her abdomen began to enlarge, she hid her condition by wrapping a bandage tightly around her abdomen. She continued to do this, obviously realizing the negative reactions she would get from the people around her, including her own family members. Of course, she was going through all of the physical symptoms, including dizziness and nausea, but she said nothing. Finally, the onset of labor pains moved her to go to a Red Cross hospital in Seoul (the equivalent of a welfare hospital in the United States), but she was too frightened to approach a doctor or a nurse. So she went into the ladies' rest room and had the baby there. Eventually, a janitor went in and found them, and the mother and child were taken to the doctor. The hospital maternity ward had a representative from an adoption agency on duty, who was alerted to the fact that an unwanted baby was available for adoption. The girl's family was notified so that they could sign the papers for the adoption, and the baby was taken by the agency. The social worker affiliated with the agency counseled the young girl for three months after the delivery. The girl decided to change schools because she was afraid that she would not be accepted by those who knew her. She continued to write to the social worker secretly after the counseling ended and inquired about her child. The social worker was impressed by the girl's concern for her baby.

If there were more recognition and acceptance by society of such births, more adequate social and health care services would be provided to such young women, and this one might have chosen to keep her baby. Here we can see the powerful negative sanction that the society exerts on young mothers having babies out of wedlock. For us in human services, social values are, therefore, a pivotal issue.

Opportunity for Unmarried Pregnancy and Adoption

Because such attitudes and social norms prohibit recognition and acceptance of premarital sexuality, the problem of pregnancy outside of marriage is very much a hidden one. Until recently, the Korean government discouraged studies of teenage pregnancy and childbirth. Consequently, empirical data on these subjects are very limited. Despite strong negative attitudes, however, more and more unmarried young women find themselves in a situation where they have to decide what to do about an unwanted pregnancy.

Most of these young women are from low-income families and work for low wages or are still in school. In a country where there are few social and health programs for teenage mothers, premarital pregnancy results in serious social, health, and financial consequences.

In Korea, young boys and girls of low-income families often move into cities after they complete the ninth grade to work in factories, stores, or restaurants. The young people work in the city to save money for their weddings or to help their families financially. Large factories have dormitories for some of their workers but cannot provide rooms for all. Those who cannot get a place in one of the dorms end up in cheap boarding-houses. A number of girls begin spending time with their boyfriends, and in many cases the boys invite them to move in rent-free if they will do laundry and cooking. This arrangement is agreeable to both parties for financial as well as social reasons. Many of these girls and boys had not had sex education. The potentially risky situation is compounded by the absence of their parents. If these youth were living at home, they would be under their parents' supervision, but because they are far from home and family, there is less pressure to conform to family and community values.

When a nonmarital pregnancy occurs, the young woman finds herself very much alone. Some teenagers get pregnant and then get married, but more give birth out of wedlock. As the traditional value system is still strong, it is a disgrace for the family if an unmarried daughter becomes pregnant. In a village or small town, the chief may feel that the incident will bring shame to the community and have a bad influence on the children, so he may put pressure on the girl to leave. In factories and workshops, both unmarried mothers and their boyfriends are often simply fired or forced to marry.

A few families, mostly of the middle-class, are willing to keep out-of-wedlock babies. In fact, the number of Korean families adopting such babies has been increasing. Social workers suspect that the adoptive families are mostly ones where the grandmother wanted to raise more children, or someone else in the family was unable to have children.

Attitudes about Marriage and Family

Published data show very low rates of premarital childbearing in Korea (Durch 1980), although the validity of these data is often questioned. There could be several reasons for reporting such low rates among young unmarried women.

Korea's experience with marriage differs even from that of other Asian countries. The literacy rate in Korea is one of the highest among these countries. Almost all young people finish middle school and high school, and many choose to go on to college. They opt for further education and postpone marriage to their late twenties (Durch 1980). In contrast, many young people in other Asian countries marry at age fourteen or fifteen, and girls experience puberty earlier. Koreans, however, consider teenage pregnancy undesirable socially, financially, and medically. Reflecting this hard-set social attitude, the average age at marriage is generally twenty-three to twenty-five years for women, and it seems it may be rising.

In Korea, there are three types of marriage: free marriages, where the couple decide that they want to be together; half-and-half marriages, where the couple exercise some control over who their future mate is but the families of the couple also have some say in the matter; and totally arranged marriages, which are still fairly popular. Why would young people in the 1990s consent to arranged marriages? In a recent survey nearly 70 percent of young and middle-aged adults in Korea were found to prefer to have their parents' consent to the selection of a prospective spouse (Sung 1987). They seem to feel safe if they conform to traditional models of marriage. In fact, most young people are still quite dependent on their families even after they marry. Parents give their children everything while they are growing up and children are, in turn, expected to take care of their parents in their old age. About 80 percent of elderly parents live with their children, even in cities (Sung 1990).

Children, mostly boys, find jobs in cities, and their parents move in with them after they set up a household. Young people feel responsible for taking care of their families and do assume this duty. If they failed to do so, the community would criticize them for being inconsiderate and selfish: the traditional ideal of filial piety is still dominant among many families (Sung 1990).

One factor that substantially affects marriage practices is the scarcity of women in the countryside. Young women prefer to live in the city because of the job opportunities, their dislike of farm work, and their desire to be near a cultural center. Consequently, for young men in the countryside it is exceedingly difficult to find wives and raise families. This has emerged as a serious concern in the country. The response of the government to this unusual phenomenon—a result of rapid industrialization—so far has been to offer incentives to young women to move out to the country.

Most families in Korea are of the traditional type, that is, two parents, children, and extended family members, but there are a few nontraditional ones as well. An example of this nontraditional family is the single-parent family with adopted children. It is now legal for a single parent to adopt and raise children, but the resulting families are considered strange.

Increasing numbers of families are adopting children, but Koreans are highly "blood conscious" and often feel uncomfortable with children who are not related by blood to their parents. Some families who choose to adopt children hide the adoption from others.

Widows with small children are looked upon favorably and are able to receive minimal financial assistance and housing at special homes for widows and children. Divorce is still rather limited and occurs most often among young people and highly educated people.

Changing Attitudes about Sexuality

In many ways, practices in Korea have become Westernized, but many of the traditional beliefs about sexuality are still in force. Dating has become widespread and is accepted by the public, including conservative parents. Much of this is casual dating, but about half of these relationships seem to lead to marriage.

A practice that is a little more controversial is young men and women living together. Parents and other adults do not like this practice, but they are in the same position as their counterparts in the West—they cannot control their children's behavior outside the home. The major variable that affects young people's habits is, in this case, the amount of control their parents can exercise.

Premarital sex is another topic that is kept very quiet. No statistics are available, so that no one really knows how widespread this practice is, but social workers and others generally know that it is occurring.

Contraceptives are readily available in Korea, both over the counter and by prescription. Minors can informally obtain these products without parental consent. The IUD was popular until the early 1970s. At that time, approximately 40 percent of women who practiced birth control used it (Ministry of Health and Social Affairs 1987). Medical problems associated with it and the necessity of consulting a doctor to obtain it were primary factors in the decline of its usage. Oral contraceptives became more popular and are today one of the methods of choice. The government encourages people to undergo tubal ligations and vasectomies, because these methods are the least expensive and the most effective. As a matter of fact, Korea has been one of the most successful countries in family planning for married adults. The government's stance toward abortion as a family planning method has also been favorable, and abortion is informally available to all who want it.

Sexuality is not often portrayed in the media because societal values do not encourage it. Newspapers and other media do not report on these subjects very frequently. This hesitancy on the part of the media reflects the taboos against public displays of or discussions about sexuality.

In recent years, sex education has been introduced in secondary schools. This new program is still in the experimental stage, and many young people do not know the facts about their own sexuality. This is due in large part to the strong popular opinion that children in school should not receive sex education, a social attitude especially evident in rural areas.

After years of successful family planning, the average age at marriage has risen and the age at first pregnancy is also somewhat late: between twenty-five and twenty-nine (National Bureau of Statistics 1986). The desired number of children has also decreased. In 1970, the number was three; now it is between one and two children. There is a difference between urban and rural communities. In cities, the number is 1.4; in the country, it is higher. Part of this is due to a preference for boys. It has been traditional for women to continue bearing children until they have a boy. Attitudes about this have changed in recent years; although some preference for boys remains, increasingly more couples see that girls are also desirable.

Services for Young Women and Children

Services to pregnant unmarried women are minimal, as described earlier. There are only four maternity homes for these women in the metropolitan Seoul area; these are sponsored by various churches and maintained by professional social workers. Partial support for these homes comes from the government, and the support will be expanded in the future.

Korea has a maternal and child health care tracking system that monitors the needs of the children and notifies the family about vaccinations and other child health matters. All women have access to prenatal care. Family planning services are offered to women in a variety of settings. All of these services are being integrated to form a comprehensive, nationwide maternal and child health care program. This program is underutilized by young unmarried or teenage mothers because of shyness in the face of negative social attitudes and/or inability to pay for the service, and the program's failure to regard these women as qualified to receive service. These factors seriously limit the program's accessibility and effectiveness.

Korea does not lack the capacity to take care of unwed pregnant women. There are many hospitals and clinics, and all of the hospitals have many doctors. But these health care systems have been hesitant to expand their services specifically for unmarried pregnant adolescents. Although they are aware of the women's great need for professional services, many health care providers seem to be caught between professional obligation and traditional influences and attitudes.

Instead, adoption services are provided to the young mothers (Sung 1985). Four adoption agencies take care of unwanted, abandoned, and lost children. Approximately 2,000 children were adopted through these agencies in 1991. The majority of these children go to homes in the United States (70%) and Europe (30%). This number is expected to decrease by 30–50 percent in the next few years. The decrease is attributed to the expanding use of family planning methods among young people and increased rates of in-country adoption by Korean families.

The need for services to teenage mothers, however, has not decreased. The number of young mothers who want to keep their babies is slightly increasing, and these young women and their babies need more services. The long waiting list of young mothers who want to enter maternity homes is indicative of this growing need.

To attack all the potential areas of dysfunction in this high-risk group of young women, comprehensive community-wide programs are needed—programs that prevent the adolescents' problems through sex education and contraception, crisis intervention when pregnancy is discovered, prenatal care and education during pregnancy, and ongoing community resource utilization (Osofsky and Osofsky 1978). Most of these girls are from families of very low socioeconomic status, and all need financial assistance, counseling, jobs, job training, access to social and health care services, and empathic support by the society (Sung 1985).

Concluding Remarks

A critical duel goes on in Korea between the dominant values in the society and the powerful changes caused by industrialization. Whether the traditional values will persist so that unmarried pregnancy will continue to be hidden and unaddressed or whether incoming forces will overwhelm the old values is a serious issue whose outcome we shall have to see.

Koreans have to envision teenage pregnancy and the problems associated with it as real problems existing within their society. They should not regard adolescent pregnancy and childbearing as abnormal or deviant or let themselves ignore the problems that youth confront in managing the transition to adult status. This perspective tends to ignore the larger social structural conditions that create the problems. Negative public attitudes will change if the problems of young people are appraised realistically and not simply attributed to individual deficiencies and pathologies that adolescent parents are believed to possess. To this end, the public must be educated about the social problems and provided with realistic assessments of the consequences of adolescent pregnancy (Siegel and Morris 1974; Klerman 1975; Bolton 1980).

These changes are within Korea's capability. In the last several decades, there has been rapid development in the areas of social and health care services in the country. However, these resources can be utilized effectively only if the traditional values and beliefs about pregnancy outside of marriage are softened or altered so that human service professionals are able to take a more compassionate approach toward these young women.

Despite the old values existing in the society, policymakers and human service professionals, such as social workers, health care providers, educators, and ministers, will have to take initiatives for positive changes. With the impetus created by these professionals, society will have to develop comprehensive programs designed to provide adequate and effective services to the young. In Korean society, young people have not been accorded priority. Family planning programs have placed emphasis on married people (Darabi et al. 1979). Organized family planning services combined with sex education must reach out to young people. Such programs must stress the risks of teenage pregnancy and offer practical advice on effective contraception.

In addition, needs for several other measures were suggested by social workers directly involved in services for the young mothers and their children (Sung 1985). They include parent education, stabilization of the family function, institution of legal sanctions against child abandonment, assistance to unwed mothers (financial aid, prenatal and postpartum care, maternity care, employment services), revision of maternal and child welfare laws to include unwed mothers and their children, education for the public on social responsibility and needs for humane and professional care for high-risk mothers and their young children, expansion of in-country adoption programs, and a more viable child care service system for the nation.

This chapter has discussed one of the most complex and nagging problems of industrialized societies. The variables underlying our concerns are the usual ones—low education, poverty, family disorganization, conservative society values, inattention by society, social environmental forces, inadequate services, and so on. These factors are closely interrelated and they all have to be tackled by the professionals and the public in a concerted manner in order to alleviate or prevent the problems of teenage pregnancy and childbirth.

Korea has been increasing its welfare programs and thus its capability to respond to the needs of the people. With steady economic growth, this process will continue. Teenage pregnancy has become a reality but not yet a large social issue in the country. However, it has become more visible as the number of young women visiting human service agencies has increased.

It will be extremely difficult and unrealistic to return to the "no-service" era from today's expanded social welfare. Young women must be provided with care and services. The long-term benefit from these services accruing to the young mothers and their children will be very valuable to Korean society.

The problems of adolescent mothers are multiple, complex, and challenging. Practitioners and researchers should continue to exchange information as to the organizational and treatment approaches that work best with adolescent clients and their children.

Koreans must study the serious approaches being taken by Americans and Europeans in order to alleviate or prevent the negative consequences of teenage pregnancy.

Teenage pregnancy is not exclusively a Western problem. In spite of the differences in culture, the crucial variables appear to be similar both in Korean and Western societies.

NOTES

1. This case was made known to the author by the social worker involved.

BRITTA HOEM

12 Early Phases of Family Formation in Contemporary Sweden

Although Sweden shares the general features of recent demographic developments with many other countries, it has been ahead of the others in most of the relevant trends (Popenoe 1987). For instance, Sweden has led the way in the decrease in marriage rates and the increase in nonmarital cohabitation (Hoem et al. 1990). Almost half of all Swedish children and two in three of first children are now born outside marriage.[1] The labor force participation of mothers with preschool children is at a record high (Layard and Mincer 1985).

At least until the early 1980s, the age at which young men and women in Sweden began their first marital or nonmarital unions dropped; and with previous childbearing patterns, this would have led to an increase in births to mothers at younger ages, as was the case in the late 1950s and early 1960s. The more recent trend, however, has been in the opposite direction. Despite the fact that young Swedish men and women continue to say they want to be parents (Nordenstam 1984; Rolen and Springfeldt 1987), young couples are in no hurry to begin childbearing. Sweden is among the many countries in which motherhood has been postponed substantially in recent decades. To start a union no longer indicates the intention to have children soon.

Instead, a new phase in the life cycle has appeared as consensual union has become a generally accepted alternative to marriage. Couples live together, often for a rather long period, without being married and without the obligations connected with parenthood. The practice of starting a union by marrying has just about disappeared in Sweden. It has also become more common that the first union is dissolved, sometimes after quite a brief period, and is followed by a new union. The strong increase in dissolutions among young cohabiting couples without children must not in itself be interpreted as a reduction in the stability of young Swedish *families,* however, for the character of early unions has changed radically. The early phases of a consensual union have largely replaced the previous practice of going steady and not the first period of a conventional marriage.

There are many competing explanations for the postponement of having the first child. The new contraceptives, improved education, and the recent changes in the status of women are some of the most frequently cited reasons. All of them have surely contributed, but at the same time there have been strong attitudinal changes about what is important at various ages in life.

Young people do not want to get tied up with all the responsibilities of child rearing as early as their parents' generation did. Many things are seen as more important than starting a family at a young age. Besides acquiring more education and establishing themselves in the labor market, youth want to earn money to spend on things they want to buy, to have time for their own leisure interests (sports, hobbies), and to travel and see the world (Rolen and Springfeldt 1987). The postponement of having the first child gives scope for early adult roles different from those of previous generations. It is the purpose of this chapter to describe and discuss such developments, particularly in the very early phases of adult life, concentrating on the period since the mid-1960s.

Our main results are based on the 1981 Swedith fertility study. In addition, we have used some data from a mail survey by Statistics Sweden in 1985 of almost 600 male and female people between sixteen and twenty-four years old. The aim of the youth survey was to get an impression of how young people viewed their future and especially the importance of family and children during the next five years.

The Role of Public Policies

In the modern Swedish welfare state, social policy is built on institutionalized reallocation of income and services, in contrast to a model of social insurance where recipients receive only what they have paid for. Perhaps more than elsewhere, priority is given to ensuring a decent level of living for everyone rather than letting market forces dictate peoples' life chances. A proper understanding of Sweden's role in this connection must take into account such particular ideological features.

In the educational system, the ambition is to give all children the same opportunity to get an education, wherever they live and whatever their social background. Compulsory school attendance has been extended to nine years; anyone who wants to may continue for another two to four years.[2] The importance of being well educated is strongly emphasized; adults are offered compensatory education so that any differences in educational level between younger and older generations may be reduced.

Labor policies aim at full employment, and great efforts are made to achieve it. As in many other countries, the unemployment rates grew in the early 1980s, particularly for young people. Therefore, special arrangements have been made to facilitate the transition from school into the labor market for this age-group. The youngest (at sixteen to seventeen years) are mainly offered more education. The unemployed at ages eighteen and nineteen are offered half-time jobs, mostly in the public sector, so that they get some work experience.[3] They are expected to spend the rest of the time looking for permanent jobs or getting more education or both. Unfortunately, it is difficult to survive on a half-time salary, and it has become rather more difficult to get ordinary full-time jobs, which now are offered more often to other age-groups (Forneng 1987). Another unexpected consequence is that the problem of unemployment has been postponed until youth's early twenties. By *international* standards, however, youth unemployment is still very low in Sweden.

Though policies are essentially based on high principles of humanist morality, Swedish public life has its own notions of what is and what is not of public concern. In particular, people's normal family life and sexual behavior are firmly considered to be in the private domain. In this, public policies' objective is to encourage unrestricted individual choice and pay little attention to procreation. Typically, sex education is a long, firm tradition in Swedish schools. Contraceptives have long been promoted openly, and the rules on abortion have always been most liberal by contemporary standards. It is easy to get married and equally easy to get a divorce. This is modified by consistently striving to defend the weaker party in any conflict of interest. Family law is being extended to do so when a consensual union breaks up, essentially introducing a modern version of common-law marriage, a concept otherwise unknown in Swedish law.

In other fields, Swedish notions about the domain and direction of public concerns can strongly guide individual choice. For instance, the country's firm public commitment to the principle of gender equality and its stress on economic activity as the proper way to achieve it are important parts of the story of women's labor force participation. Any woman may choose to be a housewife and some do, but the tax and wage structures and other practical and financial inducements make few choose this option. Individual taxation (introduced in 1971) has changed the cost-benefit calculations for families dramatically. It has become more advantageous for a wife to work, even short hours at a low-paid job, than for her husband to work overtime. This is true also for working-class families. Attitudinal changes have followed these developments and have accelerated social change. There has been a massive shift in the value of the role of housewife, to such an extent that women will no longer regard the housewife's status as equal to that of a paid jobholder.[4] Gender equality is largely interpreted as "sameness" between women and men; you cannot be an "equal" if you are a housewife, no matter what your family obligations entail.

It is part of the system that these policies have been backed by strong efforts to facilitate the dual paycheck arrangement. Sweden has invested heavily in public child care facilities and is working toward overcoming the shortage that still occurs in many places. The goal of equalizing the roles of men and women both in the labor market and at home is by no means restricted to Sweden, but we believe that the policies toward this end have been more determined in Sweden than in many other countries.

Family Policy in Contemporary Sweden

During the 1960s and 1970s, Swedish women became integrated as workers in the labor market. Most women with young children work part-time (Sundstrom 1987; Bernhardt 1988), and they still have the main responsibility for domestic work and child care. Getting fathers to participate more actively in family chores has become an important political issue since the early 1970s. A long step in this direction was taken in 1974 when fathers became entitled to parental leave from their jobs after the birth (or adoption) of a child, with compensation for the corresponding loss of earnings. (Mothers have had that right since 1955.) Parents have a legal right to choose freely which of them should stay home to take care of the newborn child, and they can decide to share the parental leave and even to spread portions of it over the years after the birth.

The Swedish scheme of parental benefits now provides a total of twelve months' leave from employment at nearly full salary and another three months' at a reduced salary. Extensions are being discussed.[5] Fathers of newborn children also have the right to stay at home for ten days in connection with the delivery.[6]

For many years, women employed in government have had the further right to take a subsequent unpaid leave of up to eighteen months after confinement and to return to the same employer. In 1979, this right was extended to all women, whoever their employer is. Even if women have no *legal* right to extend the leave any further, many employers permit even longer periods. Since 1980, absence from work with normal pay to look after sick children amounts to sixty days per year and per child for both parents together. Both parents also have the right to reduce working hours to 75 percent of full time (with a corresponding cut in pay) as long as they have children under eight. All parents have these rights irrespective of their marital status.

Swedish fathers use their newly won rights only to a limited extent, however. It is still mostly the woman who stays at home and takes care of a newborn child. To some extent this must be a natural consequence of the practice of breast-feeding, but even after the child is weaned, relatively few fathers take parental leave. Certainly, a main reason for this is the slow change in ingrained male attitudes and role patterns.[7] In addition, many women are unlikely to want to give away part of this rare period in life when they are paid not to work but to spend time with their children.

On the other hand, most fathers use their ten days of leave with pay in connection with a delivery, and men stay at home to take care of sick children almost as often as the women do.[8] Sandqvist (1987) explains this as role sharing and equality in which men will willingly engage, whereas an extended parental leave would imply role reversal, which is harder for most men to accept. Furthermore, social pressure to conform to traditional role patterns may be exerted on women. A mother who returns to work even three or four months after delivery, say, may be met by a great deal of surprise and perhaps some negative reactions from friends and colleagues, female and male.

In working life regulations to promote women's equality with men, Sweden is one of the most egalitarian societies in the world, although there is still a gap between ideology and reality.[9] Government policies have played an important role in maintaining Swedish natality at a level that rates quite highly in Western Europe.

The Emergence of a New Style of Living Together

One of the most dramatic sociodemographic changes in the past twenty years has been the postponement of marriage. As we have noted, Sweden has been at the forefront of this development. The decline in marriage rates does not imply that more young people prefer not to live in partner relationships nowadays; in fact, the situation is quite the reverse. At least as far back as our population statistics go (and Sweden has them going back many years) the proportion of young people who live in conjugal unions has never before been so high as in the late 1970s. But instead of marrying, people today just move in together without any kind of registration and in most cases without any kind of contract.

To start a union without marrying is not a new phenomenon in Sweden.[10] It goes back more than a century. We do not really know how common consensual unions were before, however, and the Swedish fertility survey of 1981 provides the first opportunity to investigate consensual unions in depth.[11] In the fertility survey, all female respondents were asked to report all the times when they had lived with a man and whether they had ever been married to him. Some women may not have reported brief childless relationships, especially in the oldest cohorts. Conversely, women in the youngest cohort may perhaps have reported rather too many relationships as consensual unions. Trost and Lewin (1978) have shown that sometimes even the partners involved in a relationship have different opinions about its character. It can also sometimes be hard to give the exact date when a consensual union started; partners often move in together only gradually. For such reasons, some of our respondents reported a consensual union only as having started during a particular winter, spring, summer, or fall, instead of in a calendar month as they were asked to do. Such possible misreporting will not change the main features of the trends observed, however.

In the oldest cohort of the fertility survey (women born in 1936–1940), more than 40 percent of those who ever started a first conjugal union (before entry into motherhood) reported that they began as cohabitants. (Because of the low visibility of the phenomenon at the time it happened, this is a surprisingly high proportion.) Most of them married rather quickly afterward, however; and durable consensual unions were relatively rare and received little public attention.

From the mid-1960s, consensual unions grew quickly in popularity and visibility. There has been a remarkable increase in the proportion of women who have chosen to start a consensual union instead of a

TABLE 12.1

Respondents Who Entered Their First Union Childless by Birth Cohort, Age, and Pregnancy Status at Entry

WOMEN BORN IN	UNDER AGE 20 (%)	PREGNANT (%)	AGE 20–21 YEARS (%)	PREGNANT (%)
1936–40	19	50	21	27
1941–45	22	38	22	28
1946–50	27	29	26	12
1951–55	36	16	27	13
1956–60	49	4	n.a.	n.a.

Source: Swedish fertility survey of 1981.
Note: Women born 1956–60 were just 20–24 years old at interview, so we do not know how many of them ever started a union before age 22.

marriage—from 44 percent of women born in 1936–1940 to 82 percent of those born in 1946–1950 to 97 percent of those born in 1956–1960.

Together with a simultaneous lengthening of the time spent in the consensual union, this increase resulted in a sharp drop in rates of first marriage. For women aged twenty to twenty-four, the rates for first marriage fell from 190 (per thousand single women per year) in the mid-1960s to less than 40 in the mid-1980s, and they are now on about the same level as those observed for single women aged thirty-five to thirty-nine. The median age at first marriage has increased by almost five years for both women and men during the last twenty years and it was 27.0 for women and 29.6 for men in 1988.

Parallel to the increased popularity of cohabitation, there were extensive other changes in union-building patterns. It became more and more common to start a union at ever-younger ages. In our oldest cohort, somewhat less than 20 percent had entered a conjugal union before age twenty, and half of them were pregnant then. Most of those pregnancies were not planned. As many as two-thirds of the teenagers who were pregnant when they started their first union reported in the 1981 fertility survey that their pregnancy came too early or was not wanted at all (Hoem and Hoem 1987).[12] In our youngest cohort (born in 1956–1960), almost half of the respondents reported that they had begun a union as teenagers and less than 5 percent of them had been pregnant at the time (table 12.1).

Early nonmarital unions spread to groups for whom starting a union had never been a realistic option before. For example, students suddenly seem to have found a type of union that suited them (Hoem 1986).

Rates of consensual union formation more than doubled among students between the cohorts born in 1936–1940 and 1946–1950. They continued to have lower rates of union formation than nonstudents, however, especially when younger than nineteen, when they mostly still lived with and were economically dependent on their parents.

With time, the implications of living together have changed. Cohabitation has become a practical living arrangement, and the first period within a consensual union has surely to some degree replaced the previous practice of going steady rather than the first period of a conventional marriage. Young people have increasingly moved in together after having known each other only briefly.

Factors Influencing the Propensity to Marry

There is little pressure to get married in Sweden nowadays. This is true even if the woman is pregnant. Remember that two out of three first-born children had unmarried parents in 1986. But some people do marry, and this section discusses what factors influence the decision to get married. We have again used data from the Swedish fertility survey. We shall compare the marriage intensities for women born in 1951–1956 with those from 1956–1960 (our two youngest cohorts) who had entered their first consensual union before age twenty-three. We follow the women for five years after entry.

The marriage intensity is the conditional probability that a couple in a consensual union will marry when it has lasted a specific length of time if they have not already married. Intuitively, it can be thought of as indicating the couple's propensity to marry at specific monthly intervals after the consensual union began. The propensity to marry is assumed to be influenced by a number of factors (regressors), such as social background, age at the start of the union, and current employment status. Our purpose is to discuss the effects these have on marriage intensity.[13]

Four of our regressors are fixed, that is, they are characteristics of a woman that do not change during the segment of her life that we study: her birth cohort, her social background, her age-group at the start of the consensual union, and whether, in the interview, she reported herself as religiously active or not.[14]

The other three covariates change with time, which means that a woman can move among the different levels of each of these factors during the period studied. Our first such covariate is the woman's current educational level in any month.[15] The next is her current number of children. We have used only two levels for this: no children (parity 0) and one child (parity 1). Women are dropped from the analyses of marriage intensities after they have become pregnant with a second child.

The last covariate is the woman's current employment status, which has seven different levels in this analysis. In any month a woman may be doing full-time work or part-time work, or be a housewife, a student, or in another status (unknown activity, unemployed, etc.). In addition, we have classified a woman as having a special employment status if she is pregnant, and another special employment status during the first year after entry into motherhood. This may be an unusual pair of "employment" statuses, but it nicely reflects behavioral changes during pregnancy and maternity leave, changes that dominate real employment status during such periods.

As can be seen in table 12.2, there has been a decrease in marriage intensities over the two birth cohorts; cohabiting women born in 1956–1960 had about 35 percent lower marriage intensities than women born five years earlier, ceteris paribus. A woman's social background had almost no influence on the marriage intensity, but, as expected, her age at entry into the union had an effect. Those who were less than eighteen years old when they started their consensual union were much less prone to marry than women who started between ages eighteen and twenty-two.

The strongest influence on marriage intensity comes from religiosity; women who reported themselves as religiously active had six times as high marriage intensities as those who did not. An earlier investigation (Hoem and Hoem 1992) has shown that religiously active women choose to marry directly more often than other women.[16] Now we can see that the relatively few of them who entered a consensual union also preferred to convert it into a marriage much oftener than other women.

There are no strong effects on the marriage intensity from the next two factors in table 12.2. Women with a low educational level had a somewhat lower relative marriage risk than other women, and cohabiting women with one child had only a slightly higher marriage intensity than childless women. It is remarkable that this difference is so small, but it must be seen in the light of the outcome on the subsequent factor in the table, namely, current employment status. Not surprisingly, pregnant women have had by far the highest marriage intensity. It was estimated as almost five times as high as for women who worked full-time and were not pregnant. (Full-time work was the most common employment status for nonpregnant women with no children, so it is the natural baseline level for this factor.)

TABLE 12.2

Relative Risks of Marriage among Cohabiting Women

FACTOR	RELATIVE RISK
Cohort born in	
1951–55	1
1956–60	0.64
Social background	
Middle and higher white collar employee	1.06
Other	1
Age at start of union	
Under 18 yrs.	0.57
18–19 yrs.	1
20–22 yrs.	1.00
Religiously active?	
Yes	6.05
No	1
Educational level	
Low	0.77
Middle	1
High	1.07
Parity	
0	1
1	1.18
Current employment status	
Full-time job	1
Part-time job	0.96
Housewife	1.17
Student	0.65
Other	0.98
Pregnant	4.89
Child less than	1.27
12 mos. old	

Source: Swedish fertility survey of 1981.
Note: Baseline levels are indicated by a relative risk of 1 (without decimals).
Time variable: Months since entry into consensual union (grouped). Entries while still childless only. Women are censored (observation is stopped) at second pregnancy, at union dissolution, 5 years after entry, and at interview.

This illustrates again that marriage formation often indicates the intention to have children soon. The second-highest relative marriage risk was found for women who had a child less than one year old. Since such a woman has parity 1 by definition, her relative risk of marrying compared to that of a childless woman in a full-time job is estimated by multiplying together the relative risk at parity 1 and the relative risk for women with a child aged less than one year, and we get 1.27*1.18 = 1.5, with one factor coming from each of the two final panels in table 12.2.[17] There is no essential difference in marriage intensity between women with full-time and part-time jobs. Women who are still in school have low marriage rates.

In the fertility survey, all women who lived in a consensual union at the interview were asked whether they believed they would eventually marry their partner sometime in the future. As many as 35 percent of the cohabiting women in our youngest cohort union (born in 1956–1960) reported that they had not even discussed this topic (Nordenstam 1984). In spite of that, only 16 percent believed that they would not marry him; 48 percent believed that they would eventually marry him; and 36 percent answered "perhaps." Presumably, at least some of these women were against the marriage as such, perhaps not in principle but simply because they did not plan to live in the current union forever. Of course, these figures cannot be used for an accurate forecast of their future marriage rates. They show, however, that although marriage was still a quite foreseeable alternative for the majority of our youngest Swedish cohabiting respondents, it belonged somewhere in their indefinite future.

The Postponement of Motherhood

The two processes—entering a conjugal union, and having children—have become more and more separated from each other, and most young people who start living together in Sweden today have probably not made any firm decision at all about when to have children. It is, however, evident from responses to questions both in the 1981 fertility survey and in the 1985 youth survey that most Swedish women and men still expect to have children, although many women now postpone the birth of their first child until their mid- or late twenties. There has been a striking decrease in the rate at which a woman of a specific age enters motherhood, and it has not been confined to the young ages. Among women born in the 1940s, about 40 percent had not had a child by the end of their twenty-fifth calendar year. The corresponding figure was some 60 percent for women born in the late 1950s. This is as far as sufficiently complete cohort data go, but the postponement is expected to continue for women born in the early 1960s as well.

Teenage mothers have become relatively rare in Sweden, and childbearing among women under eighteen has almost disappeared. If we compare age-specific fertility rates for single-year age-groups, we find that it is not more common for a woman of nineteen to have a child than it is for a woman of thirty-seven.[18]

As a consequence of the propensity to marry in connection with child-bearing, married women have much higher first-born rates than women in consensual unions. Etzler (1988) has shown that the first-birth rates for both married women and women in consensual unions have been remarkably stable over the last couple of decades. Furthermore, the marital first-born intensities are almost the same, whether a woman has lived in a consensual union for a couple of months only or for several years before marriage.

Results of an intensity regression for first borns are shown in table 12.3. To avoid the problematic causal relations involved in marriages formed in connection with childbearing, we have included all women as long as they live in their first union, whether they cohabit or are married, and have not included a civil status indicator among the regressors. To avoid anticipatory effects of an impending first birth on the employment status, we "froze" it at its level seven months before any first birth.

Women born in the late 1950s have had about 30 percent lower first-birth rates than women born five years earlier. This decrease has mostly been concentrated at short durations of the union, mainly as a consequence of the fact that a diminishing number of women were pregnant already when they entered the union.

Note that the first-birth rate *increases* with age at union formation. This is what one would expect in a society where young people want to postpone their first births to somewhat higher ages, but it is really a new pattern. Earlier, a low starting age always meant a high first-birth intensity, as it has in most contemporary societies.

According to this model, the woman's educational level was a very important factor, in contrast to the case for either marriages or dissolutions. At these rather young ages, the first-birth rates decrease strongly with an improving educational level, and the more highly educated women had first-birth rates that were only about a third of those for women who had not had much post-compulsory schooling.[19] At the same time, students had lower first-birth rates than jobholders, as one would expect.[20] Students have lower fertility than jobholders, and the very few women who reported themselves as having been housewives before they started childbearing had a very high fertility.

The postponement of the first birth is connected with some remarkable changes in norms and attitudes. Respondents in the 1981 fertility survey who were as much as twenty-five to twenty-nine years old, lived in a union, and were sure they wanted children, but had still not borne a

TABLE 12.3

Relative Risks of First Birth, All Women Living in a First Marital or Nonmarital Union

FACTOR	RELATIVE RISK
Cohort born in	
1951–55	1
1956–60	0.68
Social background	
Middle and higher white collar employee	0.69
Others	1
Age at start of union	
Under 18 yrs.	0.79
18–19 yrs.	1
20–22 yrs.	1.15
Educational level	
Low	1.51
Middle	1
High	0.54
Current employment status	
Full-time job	1
Part-time job	0.98
Housewife	2.97
Student	0.75
Other	1.28

Source: Swedish fertility survey of 1981.
Note: Baseline levels are indicated by a relative risk of 1 (without decimals).
Time variable: Months since entry into first union (grouped). Entries at parity 0 only. Women are censored at dissolution, 5 years after entry, and at interview.

child were asked why they had not had a child yet. The most common answer was that they had not yet felt mature enough. Similarly, young male and female respondents in the 1985 youth survey were more interested in getting ahead in their jobs and in earning money to buy what they wanted or develop their leisure activities than in starting a family and having children. Evidently, a new age-grading of young adult roles has been introduced.

Demographic Trends in the 1980s

So far we have mainly discussed demographic trends up to about 1980, the period covered by the fertility survey. After that, data limitations restrict our opportunity to study developments in depth. It seems, however, that they have proceeded in almost the same way as before. The postponement of marriages has continued, and age-specific fertility rates among younger people have stayed very low. On the other hand, Sweden has had a remarkable minor rebound in the total fertility rate, namely, from a low of 1.61 in 1983 to a temporary high of 2.13 in 1990. Younger ages have hardly been involved at all. The fertility recuperation is concentrated in ages twenty-five to thirty-five.

The development of early union formation is more uncertain. For the late 1970s, we have found signs of decreasing rates of union formation in the low twenties, particularly among students (Hoem 1986) and geographically concentrated in the major cities (Hoem 1984). Vogel (1986) has reported that young Swedes increasingly tended to stay longer with parents in the early 1980s than before. The census of 1985 also shows a diminishing number of young cohabitants as compared to 1980. As we have discussed, unemployment rates grew during the early 1980s, especially among young people, and it became more difficult for some groups to become established in the labor market and obtain a stable adequate income. At the same time, the housing situation deteriorated and rents escalated, especially in the cities. All things taken together, it is plausible that the reversal in young cohabitation was mostly a consequence of the worsening economic climate during the 1980s. There are no indications of changes in attitudes toward early cohabitation.

Discussion

Surely the advent of modern contraceptives, the increased availability of abortion, the improvements in education, and the development of women's roles and status have all affected childbearing. They should be seen in the context of a flow of many behavioral changes where each factor helped induce, and was induced by, other developments in a dynamic of interaction that defies any one-factor explanation. A drift in norms and attitudes is deeply involved in this process and may well be among its most long-lasting consequences. Take the introduction of the IUD and the pill, for instance. In principle, Swedes really knew how to avoid unplanned childbearing long before modern contraceptives were introduced, but the new devices, and the quick acceptance of abortion as a backup, went along with a new level of public and individual consciousness concerning the importance of planning each child. A new morality has developed that allows chance less scope and stresses bringing children into this world only after deliberate and responsible decision making. Swedish sex education and the media use a humanistic rhetoric to emphasize strongly the responsibilities of parenthood that must both have reflected and helped induce much of the postponement of entry into motherhood.[21]

The role of improved education and female participation in the labor force should be seen with similar detachment. Most young women in contemporary Sweden surely see themselves as permanent members of the labor force, even when they have small children.[22] They will also want to establish entitlement to the sizable income-related maternity benefits that are part of the system. This makes it almost necessary for a woman to complete her education and achieve a firm foothold in the labor market *before* she has her first child. In most cases, however, this need not take long. Most Swedish women complete their schooling as early as eighteen and nineteen,[23] which is long before normal childbearing age, and it takes less than a year to be entitled to the maternity rights that accompany a permanent job.[24] Furthermore, most women do not hold career-oriented jobs anyway.[25] The Swedish labor market is strongly sex segregated, so on the job most women do not "compete" with men but with other women in about the same situation as themselves. Instead of interpreting the substantial periods that women spend in the labor force before they become mothers as the time needed to establish their careers, it is more plausible to see it in reverse and to regard paid work as a natural activity for a woman who does not want to start parenting at a young age. This does not mean that work can be regarded as some sort of pastime nor that women consider their jobs as of secondary importance. For most women, it has become a self-evident right to be in the labor force, and other alternatives to working or studying are surely not considered seriously at this stage in life. Most working fertility survey respondents reported that they appreciated having paid employment (Nordenstam 1984), and the reasons given vary by educational level in a manner that supports our interpretation. Almost 70 percent of respondents with at least some university education said that the content of their jobs was its most positive feature. Only about 20 percent of the respondents with little more than compulsory education gave that response, and social contact with their workmates was the positive job aspect mentioned most often in this group. In modern Sweden, having a job gives a young woman legitimacy, status, and income, and allows her to pursue leisure interests that would be severely curtailed by motherhood. In such circumstances, childbearing becomes a matter for a later stage, a matter that is certainly seen as part of a full life but one that is easily and responsibly postponed until the time is ripe.

NOTES

I am grateful for the hospitality that I have enjoyed at the Center for Demography and Ecology of the University of Wisconsin—Madison during my work on this paper and wish to acknowledge computer support from the National Institute of Child Health and Human Development Center Grant HD 05876. Many discussions and much editorial advice from Jan M. Hoem have been greatly appreciated. Editorial advice from Peggy Rosenheim and Mark Testa has been helpful as well. I also wish to acknowledge the inspiration from recent papers by Siim (1987) and by Davis, Demeny, Keyfitz, Presser, Preston, and Westoff in the volume edited by Davis, Bernstam, and Ricardo-Campbell (1986).

1. These "illegitimate" children are almost always born to parents who live together in a nonmarital union. Childbearing by single women has decreased in Sweden over recent decades (Bernhardt and Hoem 1985).

2. All children in Sweden are offered the same education. There are almost no private schools, and even at the university level there are no tuition fees.

3. These jobs are paid for by the government.

4. Bjerén (1981) has found that women have come to regard market work as an obligation and the housewife's occupation as socially devalued.

5. Some groups have long advocated that fathers should be forced to take a share of parental leaves, but this has not met with sympathy in leading political circles.

6. During these ten days both parents can stay at home at the same time, which is not the case for the other periods.

7. The statistics show that the proportion of men utilizing this right increases with the woman's salary (Rolen and Springfeldt 1987). At the same time we know that women with a higher education (which means a higher salary) often are more job motivated and find their jobs more interesting than women who have less education. The latter group of women often report that the social contacts they have at work are more important for them than the content of the job itself (Nordenstam 1984). Men who want to use the parental leave sometimes meet with negative reactions from supervisors and workmates (Hwang et al. 1984). Sandqvist (1987) discusses fathers' parental leave possibilities in more detail.

8. The fact that these ten days are not transferable to the mother may be part of the explanation, but both parents are surely motivated by the opportunity to share a profoundly vital experience as well.

9. Everyone is not equally enthusiastic at the implementation of the regulations. See Calleman et al. (1984) for case studies and Gustafsson and Lantz (1985) for statistical documentation. See also Abukhanfusa (1987).

10. For references, see Hoem (1985). See also Wikman (1937).

11. Most of the empirical results of this paper have been based on the data from this survey (Arvidsson et al. 1982; Lyberg 1984; World Fertility Survey 1984). It contained 4,223 usable records from female respondents of each marital status. The respondents were born in 1936–1960. A wealth of information was obtained, including their childbearing histories, cohabitational and marital histories, and a month-by-month employment history beginning at age sixteen.

12. No doubt this is a minimum figure. The reports were about pregnancies

started twenty years before the interview. Presumably, any misreporting would tend to be in the direction of underreporting undesirable circumstances.

13.   This is done by hazard or intensity regression methods, which have become common in investigations of the simultaneous effects of several factors on the event selected for study. Our basic time variable is the number of months elapsed since entry into the consensual union. We have used only categorical covariates (regressors) and a piecewise constant baseline intensity (time grouped data).

14.   Only about 5 percent of all women in the fertility survey reported themselves as religiously active. An earlier investigation on dissolutions from this data set showed that the factor had a strong influence on the dissolution risks (Hoem and Hoem 1992, in press).

15.   It has become rather common for women to continue to further their education during the early phases of a consensual union. Therefore we have used a time varying covariate to pick up changes in educational level during our study period.

16.   Among women born in 1951–1955, 69 percent of the marriages were not preceded by a cohabitation among the religiously active women, compared to just 6 percent among other women.

17.   In the model of that table, the parity 1 factor of 1.18 represents the relative marriage intensity of cohabiting mothers (of one child) who neither married during pregnancy nor shortly after childbearing.

18.   These figures are from 1986, which was a typical recent year.

19.   At the life segments studied, the respondents of our two youngest cohorts were under twenty-seven years old, and most were under twenty-four. According to Etzler (1988), the effect of educational level is *reversed* at higher ages.

20.   Relatively few women have had time to attain a high educational level and to start a union simultaneously at these young ages. Those who have done so have spent a substantial part of their time within the union studying. Of all the time that highly educated women had spent in a first union, 40 percent was reported as periods when they were studying. Together these factors would produce very low first-birth rates.

21.   This does not mean that there is complete fertility control in the population. Even in our youngest cohort, every third fertility survey respondent who had become a mother before age twenty-three while in a consensual union reported that the child was born too early or was not wanted at all. (The figure refers to women who were not pregnant when they entered the union, which means the great majority.) This cohort was born in 1956–1960, so the respondents in question had their first children in the late 1970s. These unplanned births do not represent such a large number of children, however, for the third is taken out of a much reduced total number of children born at those young ages.

22.   Women on maternity leave remain members of the labor force by definition.

23.   According to our analysis of the 1981 fertility survey (Hoem and Hoem 1987), a smaller proportion of the time available at ages eighteen and above was spent studying among respondents in our youngest cohort than among those born just five years earlier. School participation culminated in our second-youngest cohort.

24.   Also, people in Sweden essentially have "tenure" in all jobs after six months.

25.   Indeed, this is one of the observations that make feminists complain about male domination. See Siim (1987).

MARGARET K. ROSENHEIM

13 Teenage Parenthood: Policies and Perspectives

Adolescent pregnancy and parenthood are widely seen as a serious social problem. Indeed, adolescent pregnancy was identified as "one of the
top domestic priorities of the Carter administration in 1978" (Vinovskis
this volume). The precise nature of the problem, however, is subject to
debate (Hayes 1987). For some members of the public, the problem is
that of early, nonmarital sexual activity. For others, it focuses on abortion. For still others, it is the welfare dependency, which accompanies
unwed parenthood for a portion of teenage mothers. Additional targets
could be mentioned. The way that the problem of adolescent pregnancy
and parenthood is formulated has consequences for public policy. Identifying "the problem" as early sexual activity, for example, highlights the
role of family regulation and can serve to sharply limit or preclude public
policy measures. By contrast, framing the problem as one of unplanned,
untimely parenthood may command responses in the public policy arena
ranging from supplying contraceptive information and materials to providing sex education and life-skills training through the schools. The
debates over problem characterization find parallels in differences of
opinion over who is responsible for taking what kind of action. In consequence, public policy on adolescent parenthood and its antecedents has
lacked focus and consistency.

In an important sense, however, these controversies over "problem" and "solution" reflect a more general and pervasive concern in our day: how to assist young people, given the fact of their extended economic and social dependency, in making the transition to adult autonomy. An inherent tension runs through social policy and family regulation in this regard. This tension besets policymakers just as it daily affects parents who struggle to guide and support adolescents' thrusts toward independence. We recognize adolescents as autonomous, responsible individuals in many respects, yet we are also aware that they are dependent, immature, and impractical. Modell and Goodman (1990:93) characterize adolescence tellingly when they speak of it as "a phase of imminence that is not quite imminent enough, of emergent adult biology that is not yet completely coordinated with adult roles, of hopes that are not yet seasoned by contact with adult reality, and of peer culture and society that mimic those of adults but are without adult ambitions or responsibilities." Adolescent parenthood reflects these contradictions; discouraging it challenges framers of social policy as well as those with a personal stake in an adolescent's well-being.

Yet the question must be asked, why is early parenthood widely regarded as a serious social problem? The "epidemic" of adolescent pregnancy is—at least for the moment—behind us (Vinovskis this volume). In addition, the social and economic consequences for young, and typically unwed parents appear to be less deleterious than had been assumed, and their children may turn out to manage better than the general public believes (Furstenberg et al. this volume). Indeed, early parenthood is interpreted by some as an "alternative life course" for poor disadvantaged teenagers desirous of having children (Burton 1990). It is seen as an acceptable strategy when relatives are available to ease the strain of parenting and assist the adolescent mother in completing age-appropriate developmental tasks, especially schooling (Hamburg and Dixon this volume, and references cited therein). What has become apparent over the 1980s is that the problem of teenage parenthood is neither so simple nor so uniformly intractable in long-term effects as previously believed.

Nevertheless, teen parenthood is seen to be "off-time" (Cohler, in press) in the sense that it increasingly precedes, and may interfere with attaining, other developmental milestones of adulthood, such as school completion, marriage, and financial independence. In addition, it is associated with poverty. When parenthood precedes economic autonomy, it may result in the welfare dependency of teen-parent households, and this is for many people another compelling reason for opposing teenage parenthood.

Today, it is largely taken for granted that young people need an extended period of development, lasting often into their mid-twenties, before they begin assuming the roles and responsibilities of parenthood. Yet negotiating this lengthy period of development is not without its complications. Not only has the period from childhood dependency to relatively independent adulthood lengthened, but the earlier onset of puberty results in what has been described as a developmental asynchrony in the attainment of the biological, legal, and social statuses of adulthood in modern society (Hamburg 1986; Hamburg and Dixon this volume). Although it is true that the simple fact of an asynchrony between biological maturity and the readiness to assume adult responsibilities need not necessarily result in elevated levels of teen pregnancies, out-of-wedlock births, and welfare-dependent households, certain aspects of contemporary life may render the personal balancing of this asynchrony of adult statuses a more difficult task than it was in earlier eras when pervasive social attitudes condemned premarital sex, out-of-wedlock childbearing, and single parenthood. The attenuation of the moral consensus on these matters has assisted a shift away from the traditional ordering of school-work-marriage-parent transitions toward novel patternings of life events. For example, marriage sometimes precedes the completion of schooling, cohabitation of singles is increasingly common, parenthood occurs in the absence of marriage, and a work career may be punctuated with spells of unemployment or schooling and with periods of part time or "try-on" jobs. Although each of these departures from the traditional pattern has generated concerns at times and resulted in an accommodation with dominant values at others, the general expectation still remains that parenthood, no matter what its order in the sequence of transitions to adulthood, will be deferred beyond the teenage years.

The question as we near the turn of the century is how public policy should address the widespread preference for deferred parenthood. Are there principles to guide the assignment of responsibility for prevention or palliation of the problem of early childbearing to adolescents, their parents, and the state? Can we accommodate, in the framing of public policy, widely divergent views and interests regarding early initiation of sexual activity, consequent pregnancy, and teenage parenthood and its aftermath? To what extent are the teenage years the appropriate focal point for intervention, or should a narrower or wider age-band be targeted? Should a welfare policy requiring employment of mothers of young children replace the earlier policy of supporting them in their care of children at home? This chapter aims to consider these issues in the context of changing social, economic, and legal conditions.

A few words of caution at the outset: a stereotype frequently pervades discussion of teenage sexuality, pregnancy, and parenthood. The image is one of a very young, black, never-married mother, living in the inner city, and at the early stages of forming a large family. This stereotype obscures a more complicated reality. Of the roughly 500,000 births annually to teenagers, the preponderance are to females eighteen to nineteen years old. They account for 60 percent of the total; adding in births to girls of 17 brings the total to 80 percent. Over two-thirds of the mothers are white, and 34 percent are married (National Center for Health Statistics 1990). As to the matter of completed family size, it is true that women who begin their childbearing in their teens tend to have larger families, by about one child on average (Hayes 1987; see also Furstenberg et al. 1987), but the significant differences previously found between cohorts of early and late childbearers in numbers of children have shrunk, particularly among blacks. While we do not have the information needed to locate teenage mothers by rural, semi-urban, or urban residence, enough data exist to dispel the notion that teenage parenthood is exclusively an inner-city phenomenon (Petersen and Crockett this volume).

Not only are teenage mothers divided along the above dimensions, but they also form two quite distinct groups according to age. Both socially and legally, they differ. Since students intending to complete high school will usually have graduated at or around eighteen, it can be argued that the focus of public policy should be on school-age adolescents since they are at risk of interrupting specific developmental tasks, education most important among them. With respect to the older group, however, the eighteenth birthday marks entry into adult status for nearly all legal purposes. Even so, some commentators advocate deferral of parenthood beyond the teenage years altogether, arguing that the case of "lost opportunities" applies after high school (Zimring this volume), and, in any event, public opinion appears to support the deferral of parenthood into the twenties (Neugarten et al. 1965).

Being Adolescent in the 1990s

Each cohort of adolescents passing through the teen years experiences a somewhat different sociocultural and economic setting in which their growing-up takes place (Buchmann 1989; Hoem this volume). Still, there are certain features of the contextual background of adolescent development that have been noticeable for some time and substantially alter the conditions of adolescents as compared, say, to those of one hundred years ago. Among them are a breathtaking shift in social mores, including sexual mores; the common prospect among today's adolescents of economic dependency extending beyond the teenage years well into the twenties; and the relaxation of the regulation of adolescent behavior by parents, community authorities, and legal institutions. Paradoxically, the lengthening of economic dependency coincides with the lowering of the age of majority and the foreshortening of social "childhood." This, as we shall see, is a source of tension for framing public policy.

The New "Adulthood" of Adolescence

Many adolescents enjoy privileges that enable them to act like adults. Their activities encompass a broader range of experiences than the sexual behavior and accompanying risks of nonmarital pregnancy and parenthood that are the focus of this chapter. There is, for example, the matter of work. A sizable proportion hold part-time jobs and thus expect a steady flow of money that is directed mainly to satisfy their personal wants, less often to augment the family's income. Substantial numbers are equipped with their own credit cards and checkbooks. Entertainment, clothing, cosmetics, and automotive parts and accessories are well-known targets of adolescent interest to which commercial enterprises cater quite specifically. There is without a doubt a large-scale teenage market.

Possession by adolescents of their own money, whether its source be earnings or allowance, positions young people in the mainstream of the adolescent society. The family understandings that empower adolescents with respect to personal expenditures reveal important concessions of adult authority; they symbolize parental willingness to allot decisional power over an area of activity prized by the young. That this parental judgment is often a deliberate endorsement of "growing up as a process" (Zimring 1982) does not diminish its concurrent significance as a contraction of the sphere of parental authority.

Money is by no means the only route to (limited) adolescent sovereignty. In many middle-class families it is customary for children to have their own bedrooms and equally customary for parents to defer to some extent to adolescents' desire to enjoy privacy therein. Access to the telephone is taken for granted pretty much across the economic spectrum. Possessing a room of one's own and a private conversational link to one's peers enlarges the adolescent's exclusive domain; couple these perquisites with the frequent availability of a car, and it may truly be said that "kids could run away from home without packing a suitcase" (Zimring 1982:45). The point is that contemporary child-rearing practices concede a wide area of private communication and decision making to adolescents and then hold them to modest account for what transpires there.

Now, as always, there are parents who are uninterested in or incapable of supervising their adolescent children, just as there are some communities and families in which meetings between boys and girls in their early to mid-teens would be unthinkable in the absence of a responsible adult presence. Still, as a general rule, it does appear that young people's social contacts are no longer as assiduously monitored as in the past.

Surely this reflects a shift in child-rearing standards as well as a marked change in the role of peer relationships, resulting in part from longer periods of education during which young people are immersed in an institution that draws them together and keeps most adults out (President's Science Advisory Committee, Panel on Youth 1974). Compared to the dominion of concern and control over youth that characterized pre-twentieth-century America (Teitelbaum and Harris 1977), the pace-setting of the peer group and the relaxation of parental oversight, with its accompanying demand for accountability, are in striking contrast to the past.

The "Sexual Revolution"

Changes in sexual behavior over the past fifty years have been sweeping. During this period there has been a notable shift in public attitudes toward premarital sex, and the widespread availability of effective and inexpensive contraceptives has granted women a far greater measure of reproductive control. These developments are international in scope, affecting a wide spectrum of industrialized countries (Jones et al. 1986). Moreover, these changes have occurred at a time of "the widest separation in human history between the timetables of biological maturation and the socially acceptable expression of sexual behavior" (Katchadourian 1990:330). Of paramount importance is the postponement of marriage. Marriage, it appears, has lost ground among young adults, not to mention teenagers. In the period 1960–1990, a steady and large increase in the proportion of never-married males and females occurred. Throughout this thirty-year span the proportion of never-married females under eighteen remained high (steady at over 90 percent), but the shift in marital status among the older teenagers and young adults is truly striking.

Now nearly all teenage women of eighteen or nineteen are never married, whereas in 1960 about one-fourth of eighteen-, and 40 percent of nineteen-year-olds had been married. Even more startling is the trend within the twenty–twenty-four-year-old cohort, where the proportion of never-married females rose from 29 percent in 1960 to over 60 percent in 1990. Thus, when examining sexual behavior among teenagers, we are effectively considering nonmarital behavior.

The shift in sexual behavior is pronounced across the entire spectrum of women fifteen–forty-four, the group traditionally defined as being of reproductive age. From 1955, when the first national survey into reproductive behavior was conducted, to 1988, the latest period for which data are available, the trend in nonmarital sexual behavior has been quite consistently upward. In 1988, 66 percent of never-married women aged fifteen–forty-four reported having had intercourse (Forrest and Singh 1990). Among teenagers, the proportion having experienced nonmarital sexual intercourse grew from 29 to 52 percent between 1970 and 1988. Not surprisingly, the data reveal differences in the pattern of activity between older teens and those under eighteen. Among eighteen- and nineteen-year-olds, about three-fourths report premarital intercourse (73% for whites, 76% for blacks), but the proportion among the group fifteen to seventeen so reporting in 1988 is hardly insubstantial (34% for whites, 48% for blacks; Centers for Disease Control 1991). Moreover, the age of first sexual experience has been dropping, a particularly sobering fact in that early initiation into sex "is associated with an increased number of sexual partners and a greater risk for sexually transmitted diseases" (Centers for Disease Control 1991:929).

It seems reasonable to assume that these upward trends are influenced by the existence of effective contraceptive measures, but besides the widely dispersed understanding that sexual intercourse can be dissociated from reproduction, other factors undoubtedly influence the onset and continuation of coitus among teenagers. The relaxation of adult oversight has already been mentioned. The absence of parents from the home, increasingly likely as mothers move into the work force, makes adequate supervision more difficult. Many children living in single-parent households (overwhelmingly headed by mothers) become aware of the sexual connotations of socializing between parents and their adult visitors. In addition, peer pressure is a major factor in defining what risks and pleasures to explore, with nonmarital sexual activity often associated with other types of behaviors deplored by adults (Jessor and Jessor 1977). Certainly today's teenagers are also widely exposed to sexually provocative films, television programs, music, and advertising. They are confronted with reports of the "nontraditional" liaisons of figures prominent in film and the mass media. They are exposed to much more frequent discussion about sexual relations, both heterosexual and homosexual. AIDS is covered by the national news media and increasingly addressed by schools and a variety of youth-serving groups.

The fact is that adolescents are, almost unavoidably, surrounded by symbols, discussions, and events containing sexual content. This much is obvious. Less well appreciated is the fact that the public messages adolescents receive are sharply conflicting: sex, as in a film or advertising, is typically portrayed as glamorous and associated with desired goals or products; sex, as linked to "early" sex, to pregnancy and sexually transmitted diseases, is presented as off-limits and "bad." Moreover, largely absent from the public representations intended for teenagers is acknowledgment of sex as an object of desire and pleasure and an intimacy to be achieved responsibly (Boxer this volume; Fine 1988). Adolescents themselves know about these aspects of sex, but they are seldom encouraged to discuss them. Discussions in the home, if they occur, are likely to be awkward.[1] Instead, communications directed at adolescents often portray sex as deviant, sometimes as sinful. Notwithstanding, the practice of premarital sexual relations is gaining ground as "normal" adolescent behavior (Katchadourian 1990).[2]

Legal Changes

Alterations in sexual behavior have not escaped the notice of lawmakers. Laws affecting family relations and sexual behavior have undergone substantial modification since mid-century, and the ambit of state authority over adolescents has shrunk. In each case, the desired goal of reformers has been the reduction of state power in recognition of claims to greater individual freedom from regulation. These claims in turn have been influenced by changing standards of personal behavior and family life. All of the changes affect the moral as well as the legal environment in which adolescents are learning and maturing.

First, the significance of marriage as an institution has declined. As unmarried cohabitation has become more common (U.S. Bureau of the Census 1991*b*) and public law has become an increasingly important source of financial protection for children and also for adults living in informal unions (Glendon 1981), the difference between the statuses and benefits conferred under legally constituted marriage and de facto relationships has diminished. This modern development is remarkably similar in direction and result among industrialized countries of the world (Glendon 1989; see also Hoem this volume). Thus, the importance of marriage, once a critical link to status, financial protection, and inheritance, has eroded considerably with easier access to divorce and, through both legislation and judicial decision, at least limited recognition to the "rights" and needs arising from de facto unions. What as recently as the mid-1950s was regarded as unthinkable has yielded to the tide of events; "the unthinkable [has become] the law. . . . So far as the legal position of unmarried cohabitants is concerned, . . . the principle that marriage is an essential prerequisite to the creation of a legally recognized family unit is 'now subject to many exceptions' " (Glendon 1989:269, referring to commentary on English law).

A second important development in law concerns its treatment of sexual relations. Until the recent past, only marriage offered an acceptable model for sexual relations, and the available sanctions for failure to conform were severe (Ingram 1987). Measures proscribing nonmarital sexual behavior offer striking evidence, to present-day eyes, of the widespread acceptance of extensive regulation over child-rearing practices and sexual behavior within families. Criminal laws against fornication, adultery, and sodomy were universal; their enforcement, however, was not.

These laws remained on U.S. statute books until challenged in the 1950s and 1960s, when legal scholars and legislators reconsidered the wisdom of regulating consenting adults' sexual activity. In a brief span of time, state by state the criminal laws of fornication and adultery were repealed. As a result, with some exceptions, the way was cleared for consenting adults to participate in heterosexual relations outside of marriage without fear of criminal prosecution (Slovenko 1983; on homosexuality, see Russo and Humphreys 1983; Glendon 1991). The resulting decriminalization of sexual behavior has signaled a milestone in the alteration of moral and legal standards; it confirms the evolution of more liberal social attitudes toward sexual practices and diverse family forms.

Practically speaking, decriminalization would rarely affect young people; it was a movement focused on adults. But when the young are enjoined to comply with values no longer displayed by their elders, the latters' admonitions may appear to adolescents to lack moral force. Nonetheless, minors are subject to the control and guidance of parents or their surrogates. Age—not surprisingly—makes a difference. But under what circumstances should the state be prepared to reinforce parental authority or insist, out of legitimate interest in the development of children and youth, on an independent claim to intervene? The climate of deregulated adult sex provided one context for reconsideration of the breadth of state authority over juvenile noncriminal misbehavior.

From the establishment of the juvenile court until the 1960s–1970s, extrafamilial regulation of juvenile sexual behavior was enforced primarily through the juvenile court. State power was invoked to curb the intransigence of juvenile "status offenders," that is, juveniles engaged in truancy, running away, persistent defiance of parental or parent-surrogate authority, and sexual "acting-out" (notably among girls; Teitelbaum and Gough 1977). Dispositions available to the court included probation, foster placement, and, not infrequently, commitment to the same custodial institutions that held delinquents. Sexually active and pregnant adolescents were found among female institutional populations.

This broad reach of juvenile court jurisdiction responded to Progressive Era dismay over the behavior of youth and the laxness of parental supervision, especially in expanding urban areas of the nation; the enumerated status offenses were seen as preludes to a more serious turning toward crime and delinquency. Then as now, reliance on the agencies of juvenile justice was selective. It appears to be "indisputable that, from the early nineteenth century to the present, the juvenile justice system has systematically singled out lower-class children for punishment and ignored middle- and upper-class youth" (Schlossman and Wallach 1980:66). This class bias and evidence of racial and ethnic bias, too, were critical factors influencing the 1960s drive for reform.

A movement to reexamine the breadth of juvenile court laws (Institute of Judicial Administration—American Bar Association, Juvenile Justice Standards Project 1977) ultimately resulted in severe retrenchment of state jurisdiction over the status offender category of children (Rosenheim 1976). Today, power over these juveniles is generally confined to emergencies and to a limited assertion of authority that is influenced by a crisis intervention model (Caplan 1964; Rapoport 1962) and restricted as to length of time and place of custody.

Thus, it appears that coercive control over juvenile sexual activities has been ruled out. And so it has, in the specific provisions of the past. But what cannot be achieved directly can sometimes be reached indirectly. For example, modern juvenile court statutes often include jurisdiction over drug offenders. Commonly, provisions include compulsory treatment and supervision of the adolescent substance abuser who, research studies tell us, is also likely to be sexually active (Ensminger 1987). It may prove difficult to maintain the replacement of state coercive intervention into adolescents' lives with concessions of autonomy over sexual and other noncriminal misbehavior. In the absence of effective parental oversight or adolescent self-regulation (which are missing in the typical juvenile status offender case), the pressure for state intervention sometimes becomes uncontainable; lessons from the earlier era of juvenile justice, however, surely tell us what a price we pay for trying to coerce people into preferred behavior (Rosenheim 1976; Zimring this volume).

Economic Dependency

Up to this point, the aspects of being adolescent under discussion affect all adolescents and their parents. Shifting standards for child rearing, the "sexual revolution," changes in the law—each influences the social order in which adolescents grow up. Although certainly their effect may vary markedly by race, class, or gender, they are factors common to the experience of parents and adolescents. With respect to the subject of economic dependency, however, the situation of disadvantaged youth deserves special consideration, for these young people often lack the resources to move smoothly from high school into full-time work. As policymakers confront the plight of early parents, they increasingly worry that the lengthening of economic dependency has a particularly debilitating effect on the transition of youth into approved family roles.

Traditionally, family formation patterns have been timed to coincide with the economic ability of the parties to establish an independent household and raise their children together. For the "truly disadvantaged" (Wilson 1987), however, the picture is far different. The persistence of high unemployment in the ghetto and the discouraging picture of future employment for the high school drop-out have consequences for both marriage and out-of-wedlock births (Testa and Krogh 1990). Among many young poor minority males there is seemingly little motivation to prevent a pregnancy; there is also little motivation (and scarcely any social pressure) to marry (Dryfoos 1988). The overall result for disadvantaged males and females, in contrast to their more fortunate peers, is that the costs of off-time, out-of-wedlock childbearing may seem no higher in the teenage years than later on. Hence, it is argued, their incentives to postpone marrying and raising children to the time of financial independence are weakened. This departure from an accustomed pattern linking childbearing, marriage, and economic autonomy is particularly troubling in an era when sexual activity has become loosened from the institution of marriage and the risk of out-of-wedlock births has grown.

In 1960, when one-half of American women married before or shortly after high school graduation (U.S. Bureau of the Census 1991*b*), school-age parenthood only slightly accelerated young women's entry into adult family roles. Now that the median age of marriage is the mid-twenties, girls' becoming parents during their teens greatly strains the capacity of existing institutional arrangements to provide for teen mothers and their children. These mothers are often dependent within their homes and without and unable to lay claim to adequate resources and supports in the process of discharging their off-time parental roles.

Public provision related to identifying and preparing for work roles is usually based in vocational high schools. Institutionally based assistance to support adolescents and young adults in the transition from high school to employment, with additional education or training en route as required, is either unavailable on a large scale or less coordinated and up-to-date than it should be (W. T. Grant 1988*a,* 1988*b*). To be sure, there are examples of innovative and useful programs and of notable individual efforts to help some young people, but the United States lacks the kind of widespread institutionalized provision for job training and placement that characterizes certain foreign nations (Rosenbaum et al. 1990).

One response to structural changes in the economy, not only in the United States but elsewhere, has been the deferral of family roles and the increasing enrollment of young people in postsecondary education as a means of becoming better prepared for a changing workplace and a changing market. Many middle-class youth ease into full-time careers by exploring, over an extended period, some combination of college and postgraduate education, internships in a wide variety of settings, avowedly service-oriented assignments in programs like Vista, the Peace Corps, teacher corps units and others, and travel, often with parental support.

One recommendation recurrent in policy circles where solutions to the plight of economically vulnerable non-college-bound youth are being sought is some kind of national service type of program (Sherraden and Eberly 1982; Moskos 1988; W. T. Grant Foundation 1988*b;* Eberly and Sherraden 1990). While reasons for advocating this approach vary, the benefits noted include educational and job-training opportunities and, on a more abstract level, the contribution of such programs to citizen education. Past accounts of military service and the achievements of the Civilian Conservation Corps of New Deal days (and its state-based analogues in the present day: Danzig and Szanton 1986) provide anecdotal evidence for the positive effect these programs have had on the development of participants' marketable job skills and workplace habits and are also encouraging in other respects. Among the latter are positive contributions to civic education, and thereby to the "vitality of democratic citizenship" (Janowitz 1983:203), and to the less lofty but nonetheless laudable goal of providing the young with temporary, socially approved activities to which modest monetary rewards attach.

To date, the development of institutional response to economic change in behalf of the disadvantaged adolescent has been piecemeal and slow in coming. There is growing recognition that something comparable to the role performed for middle-class youth by higher education and a variety of informal educational and service opportunities is sorely needed.

Managing the Future

At the outset, in considering directions for future public policy, it is important to recognize its limitations in affecting the level of teenage parenthood. Parents' values and the context they provide for their children's growing up are crucial influences on adolescent conduct (Hogan and Kitagawa 1985). The environment of the schools and the neighborhood and the "tone" of an adolescent's peer group are important sources of norms and self-regulating habits. Moreover, the contributions of public policy to the prevention of parenthood are further limited by the fact that the majority of teenage births occur to mothers who are eighteen and nineteen and thus beyond the reach of certain legal restrictions and youth-embracing institutions that affect the lives of younger adolescents.

Deferral of Parenthood

Nonetheless, public policy can frame a constructive approach to assisting adolescents to postpone entry into a life-changing role: raising a child. The overriding goal should be the deferral of parenthood past the age of legal majority and, preferably, after economic autonomy has been attained. While there will be individual cases—and perhaps whole communities—in which teenage parenthood is acceptable or even seen to be desirable for young people who have not completed the other transitions to adulthood, these are exceptions that prove the rule. Today, the prevailing view is that the lengthening period required for transitions—time spent in schooling, in becoming directed and moderately secure in work roles, in clarifying personal priorities for social and family life—dictates deferral of parenthood beyond the age of majority as the prudent course.

An advocate of deferring parenthood risks vulnerability to the charge that this prescription is skewed to middle-class circumstances and opportunities; it may not be functional for many economically disadvantaged adolescents. Burton (1990), writing from her ethnographic research on a community of poor black families, suggests that they "may construct family timetables that [permit] transitions to culturally defined family roles at younger ages. . . . For families in which teenage childrearing is normative, the age period defined as 'adolescence' could begin much earlier, at around 9–10 years of age, and end much sooner, at age 13 or 14." Such families may deem adolescence to end with the attainment of menarche, sexual experience, and greater participation in household management and the supervision of younger children (126).

Nevertheless, as a reliable strategy the alternative life-course crucially depends upon the existence of caretaking support (Testa chap. 6, this volume). Typically the source of support is the mother of the teenage mother, but there is reason to believe that this resource will be in shorter supply in future. The current generation of grandmothers is better educated and, having limited their fertility, younger upon completing childrearing than their counterparts in previous generations. For some, at least, the prospect of helping to raise yet another generation of children is unappealing and can give rise to friction between the grandmother and her adolescent daughter (Burton and Bengtson 1985; Brooks-Gunn and Chase-Lansdale 1991). At the same time, the identification of the alternative life-course strategy has prompted reexamination of previous claims (cited in Geronimus and Korenman 1991: abstract, nonpaginated) that teenage childbearing is "irrational behavior that leads to long-term socioeconomic disadvantage for mothers and their children." To the contrary, it has been proposed that it "may be a strategic, collective response to the constraints imposed by poverty," a reflection of "opportunity costs . . . that appear to be lower where teenage childbearing is common than in settings where it is less common" (Geronimus and Korenman 1991; see also Hamburg and Dixon this volume).

Recognizing that an alternative life-course strategy may be functional in certain contexts need not, however, undermine the case for postponement of parenthood. Rather, it serves to remind us of the diversity of family formation patterns and of the need to consider the functional purposes they serve whenever we embark on making public policy. Of the alternative life-course strategy, Burton, for example, acknowledges that adolescent childbearing violates "expected behavior in most black families and can produce negative outcomes," but goes on to say that "early childbearing may be perceived as a viable option that fosters individual growth, family continuity, and cultural survival in an environment in which few other options for enhancing development are available"

(Burton 1990:123, 124). It is to these "other options" that attention must be directed.

Improving Life Options

There is general agreement that the prevention of teenage pregnancy requires more than the provision of sex education courses and contraceptive supplies. At the same time, individuals concerned about the problem of teen childbearing are agreed on its close association with poverty and low basic skills. Data from the 1982 National Longitudinal Survey of Youth reveal that sixteen- to nineteen-year-old girls whose family income was below the poverty line and whose basic skills were below average "were five to seven times more likely to have become mothers than girls with average or better skills and not from poverty families" (21%–23% compared to 3%–5%; Dryfoos 1990:75). It is worth noting that these findings hold for whites, blacks, and Hispanics without significant differences; in each instance girls who fared better were far less likely to be parents. The implications of these data suggest a need to address both basic educational preparation and the consequences of poverty. As Dryfoos notes, findings like these demonstrate "the validity of pregnancy intervention programs that seek to expand the opportunity structure for these disadvantaged youth" (Dryfoos 1990:75–76).

More and more, programs directed to teenagers have sought to incorporate features that are intended to enhance the life options of the adolescent population served. Experience with pregnancy prevention activities has also underscored the necessity of "putting the boys in the picture" (Dryfoos 1988). Since programs are generally located in poor neighborhoods, the targeted group presumably will benefit from various kinds of assistance. Certain forms of help directly erase financial barriers by providing services and supplies that may otherwise be unaffordable, but as the focus of program broadens to include, for example, school improvement or mentoring objectives, other strategies assume greater importance. The desire to enlarge the future options of adolescents viewed to be at risk of pregnancy has led to expansion of clinic missions to create multiservice, community-based prevention programs and to community efforts to encourage new approaches to improving school performance and sponsoring preparation for and placement in employment (Hayes 1987; Hofferth 1991).

Besides prevention programs, a number of organized activities deal with teenage parents. Parenting and child development interventions and extension of service to teen fathers are among them (Hofferth

1991). The form of these programs varies; many of the services provided to parents parallel the preventive measures available to teenagers at risk (Hayes 1987). Indeed, considerable tension can develop within a given program between serving the goals of prevention and giving help to already pregnant teens or to young parents (cf. Vinovskis 1988*a*).

Service to this teenage population has not been free from controversy. Sex education proposals have attracted dissidents, and opposition to contraceptives and abortion increases when minors are the intended recipients of service. It is not surprising—given the differences in perspective among adolescents, parents, doctors, community leaders, and the policymaking constituency regarding issues related to nonmarital sex—that making rules for this area is a controversial business.

Opinions differ on whether minors should be able to secure contraceptives and abortions on their own, independent of parents who normally control decisions regarding medical care; here potential conflict involves a struggle between the adolescent, parents, and the state. Parental notification and consent requirements are a sore point of dispute. At the moment state laws differ considerably as to a minor's right to make abortion decisions and, where the right is qualified, as to the degree of involvement of her parents and the juvenile court (Gittler et al. 1990). Given the tenor of recent United States Supreme Court decisions, it is hazardous to predict future directions.

Notwithstanding, the appeal to public health considerations eases controversy—a bit. One example concerns AIDS, the other the high risk level associated with inner-city adolescent pregnancy and parenthood. The AIDS case is straightforward. The public recognizes a fatal disease transmissible through sexual relations. Preventing AIDS is in the public interest. Measures to do so can be likened to those long accepted for venereal diseases or alcohol and drug abuse. In these, public health considerations have won out over the usual respect shown parental authority, which is typically in control of the medical treatment of minors (Gittler et al. 1990; cf. Gamson 1990). Analogizing AIDS to accepted public health prerogatives has led a number of communities to establish condom distribution programs within the schools. These decisions, initially accompanied by an outcry of protest in some places and often adopted by close vote, seem to be surviving.

The public health agenda also has room for the phenomenon of inner-city adolescent parenthood. The early concern about an "epidemic" of adolescent pregnancy (Vinovskis this volume), the continuing alarm about excessively high rates of infant and maternal mortality in these neighborhoods, the numbers of low-birth-weight children with physical and cognitive deficits—all these provide scientific justification for intervening. Provision of such services as counseling, child care and parent training, family planning advice, and well-baby clinics (Schorr 1988) has recently been supplied in school-based clinics (Dryfoos 1988; Kirby 1991). Although controversial initially, these clinics are generally supported by the residents surrounding the chosen sites.

In sum, many pregnancy- and parenting-related and "life option" services are being provided to teenagers. Admittedly, coverage by these programs is limited, both within targeted areas and between regions of the country, and evaluation of their effects is sparse, though growing (Marsh 1991), but greater attention to enhancing life options is demonstrable. While certainly this expansion of service goals for teenagers at risk of or already experiencing pregnancy is laudable, one may ask whether development of life options is best undertaken in connection with programs having a specific focus on teen sexuality, pregnancy, and parenthood. Does this effort deserve attention in its own right? Consideration of this question will be deferred to the conclusion.

The Welfare Issue

It is through provisions surrounding welfare dependency that the state most substantially affects the lives of poor unwed teenage mothers. By "welfare" we refer primarily to the federal-state program of Aid to Families with Dependent Children (AFDC), but the term often also subsumes poverty-related programs like Medicaid, food stamps, and housing subsidies. Eligibility for AFDC turns on the facts of poverty and the mother's status; divorced, deserted, widowed, and unwed mothers are the major categories covered. Contemporary concern over never-married mothers on welfare stems largely from two developments: the discovery that a substantial proportion of never-married mothers who begin childbearing in their teens are on welfare for lengthy spells (estimated at between 40% and 50% of the rolls at any given time: Ellwood 1988) and a change in the roles of middle-class women, leading to altered social expectations about mothers working outside the home. These two factors, combined with a continuing high level of expenditures under AFDC, have stirred decision makers to reassess the program and make some important revisions, enacted in the Family Support Act of 1988.

Unwed motherhood has always drawn critical attention, and the fear that, failing adequate parental resources, the child's support would fall upon the public has often been pronounced. AFDC was not intended to be a major source of support for never-married mothers; it was expected to be a transitional measure, due to "wither away" as the social insurance program of Old Age and Survivors Insurance matured (Steiner 1971; Patterson 1986). Instead, the AFDC rolls have grown, and its recipient population is now dominated by never-married mothers (Congressional Budget Office 1990:46, table 10).

Recently responding to a "reform consensus" on the issue of welfare dependency (Handler and Hasenfeld 1991), Congress, through the Family Support Act, has addressed the problem in several ways: by improving child support collection procedures (a subject beyond the scope of this essay); by tightening up on the mandatory work and training provisions intended to transform economically dependent mothers into paid workers; and by restricting head-of-household status for teenage *minors,* thus targeting a possible incentive to start families and live on their own (Handler 1987–1988). Both the latter two provisions, and the strengthening of child support requirements, reflect a "social contract" model of public assistance, with implications for eligible minors as well as adults. This model rests on the belief that the state and the recipient of aid have mutual obligations, the state to provide for the poor, and the recipient to demonstrate appropriate behavior in addition to need (New York State Task Force on Poverty and Welfare 1986; Mead 1986). It derives from a growing consensus among policymakers that more should be demanded of the welfare recipient. Job training and placement and at least some support for education should be made available to the recipient, who, in turn, is expected to make efforts to become self-supporting over time.

Such a goal fits with the substantial increase in mothers of young children in the labor force, where their presence lends credibility to a reversal of the original underlying premise of AFDC, namely, that the state should support needy mothers to stay at home and care for their children. This policy has changed; from the day that job training and placement were mandated, social policy shifted to encouraging the entry of adult recipients into employment, and by doing so implicitly challenged the importance of an ongoing maternal presence in the home during the preschool and school-age years of childhood.

The question here is what a social contract model means for teenage mothers. The younger ones among the group are, after all, required to attend school. Consistent with the requirement under the Family Support Act that older mothers of children three years and older (or one year old, at state option) enroll in training or work, this statute also mandates attendance at school or training for younger mothers, thus promoting development of skill and knowledge that will facilitate their future labor force participation. Wisconsin's Learnfare provides an example of this type of welfare reform, requiring that "*all* teenagers (thirteen through nineteen years of age) who are included in an AFDC grant (both parents and children) must be enrolled in school and meet strict attendance standards . . . unless they have graduated from high school or have received some form of equivalency diploma" (Corbett et al. 1989:1 (emphasis added); cf. Jackson 1989). Learnfare is best regarded as a variant of the work and training programs now mandated for adult welfare recipients on AFDC, with an emphasis on sanctions rather than services in one state that has been studied; failure to comply entails a reduction in family benefits (Handler and Hasenfeld 1991).

The changes enumerated above have attracted wide approval. They are intended to lead to work for recipients who have completed high school, as probably most mothers of eighteen and nineteen will have done, or to Learnfare types of programs for younger recipients of AFDC. Indeed, Handler and Hasenfeld (1991) speak of a reform consensus that enjoys diverse and broad support. It centers on reciprocal obligation (the "social contract"), work, family, education, and increased latitude for the exercise of state discretion (201). Taken at face value, the consensus seems reasonable enough. The current emphasis on work assumes that it is both legitimate and desirable to expect work force participation from females on AFDC who are, by definition, mothers of "dependent" children. The fact that countless women not on welfare carry these dual responsibilities for work and child care is brought forth to support this position.

Two concerns may be noted. One relates to the question of personal judgment. Most women in the labor force make a choice to enter paid employment. Although financial stringency may be a major motivation, they nonetheless enjoy a freedom to balance preferences and evaluate domestic duties that is denied AFDC recipients. Mothers often resolve the tension between job and home by working part-time. Why is the welfare policy favoring work not put forth as a matter of choice? In a number of states work programs are oversubscribed; there are more volunteers than the state's welfare department can handle. Both for efficiency's sake and for the intrinsic value of offering mothers choice over what every mother acknowledges to be a strenuous balancing act between demands of home and workplace, choice seems to have merit.

A second concern relates to the difficulty of operating or monitoring large-scale work, training, and educational programs that evidence an understanding of each recipient's skills and motivations on the one hand, and sophisticated knowledge of employment possibilities on the other. To achieve job placements with the promise of stable employment calls for at least some degree of individualized decision-making, a task that the typical state public aid bureaucracy cannot readily perform. State and local bureaucracies, functioning under the rigorous requirements of political and fiscal accountability, may be unable to fulfill the individualization criterion. Perhaps only if protected by having the status of demonstration projects, or by being under the shelter of politically invulnerable leaders, can such individualized and therefore labor-intensive services flourish. Otherwise, state agencies, under intense pressure to demonstrate numerical success by moving recipients into work and training programs, will inevitably routinize and mass-produce decisions, hence subjecting recipients to rote investigation of their circumstances and to pressure to move into "slots" quite inappropriate for their talents. In operation, bureaucracy's efforts may work quite unfairly.

In sum, if the goals of work—and the prospect of financial independence for welfare recipients—are to be taken seriously, the administration of these programs must also be taken very seriously and (one suspects) funded at considerably higher levels, as several commentators have observed (Lynn 1989; Maxfield 1990). States have shown it can be done at times and in specific localities (Gueron 1990), but will the game appear to be worth the candle? Past practices at the local level suggest that on-line administrators may be dubious: "they have repeatedly preferred the manipulation of the gates [to eligibility] and the amount of direct cash relief rather than setting the poor to work" (Handler and Hasenfeld 1991:197; Rosenheim 1966).

Past experience, however, is not necessarily a guide to future practice. Within the ranks of liberals and conservatives alike there is grave disquiet over the costs of welfare and its use as income to support family formation by impoverished nonmarried parents. At the same time, the contemporary alliance behind a movement to stress responsibility for family and self-support is an uneasy one. It combines liberals and conservatives and yokes together those who desire to impose severe deterrent measures with advocates of Learnfare and the work and training programs who see in these activities means to better prepare poor youth and adults for self-sufficiency. As long as the reform consensus holds, the current emphases of welfare policy may well prevail since the "adjudication" of inconsistencies between liberal and conservatives will most often occur at state or local level where implementation practices give specific content to the rhetoric of consensus. Yet, if history is a reliable guide, it is highly likely that in the implementation of these welfare reforms the strategy of sanctions will predominate over the provision of service and opportunity. (See, for example, the discussion of education reform in Handler and Hasenfeld 1991).

Age as the Focus of Policy

Adolescence is an awkward phase of life for all concerned. It is inevitably awkward for adolescents and far from a comfortable phase for parents and other authority figures. But it is a necessary phase. In a diverse and somewhat fluid society that prizes individualism and personal freedom, it takes time for young people to learn the ropes and fix upon their goals and ways to reach them. The rules of personal behavior are not all that clear; neither are they uniform.

In our time, many old markers of status have disappeared, and with them a degree of certainty about acceptable conduct. But age as a signal of status survives. Age grading offers a useful approach to marking the boundaries of social problems and limiting the scope of policy response. As a reference point for framing interventions to prevent or contain adolescent pregnancy and parenthood, age boundaries appear to be eminently sensible. They reflect the social judgment that childbearing in the teen years is off-time. They have the great advantage, moreover, of facial neutrality, for using age to set policy targets avoids usage of more controversial criteria.

But there are drawbacks to this approach. For one thing the teenage years may present a superficial commonality, but they comprise, on closer inspection, a wide spectrum of development achievements and tasks. Although dramatic biological changes usually occur in early adolescence, cognitive development is incomplete until later in adolescence. Psychosocial tasks, many of which are introduced by the transition into junior high school, require new repertoires of behavioral response (Hamburg 1986; Petersen and Crockett 1986). Cognitively, biologically, legally, socially, experientially, there is little commonality between females (and males) of thirteen and those at the upper reaches of the teens.

A more important shortcoming to this approach is the danger that emphasizing age will obscure needs that transcend age boundaries. Take the case of the risks of infant and maternal mortality and morbidity associated with teenage pregnancy and childbirth. Evidence of the 1960s and 1970s pointed to a higher mortality rate among teenage mothers and their infants and to a higher than average rate of developmental deficits among children born to very young mothers (Moore and Burt 1982). Whereas there is no doubt regarding an *association* between the young age of the mother and poor health outcomes for both mother and child, for several years debate has surrounded the reasons for this finding. The now prevailing consensus is as follows: "Although a relationship between an early first birth and the child's health at birth has been found, this appears to be a result of less than adequate prenatal and perinatal care rather than biology, since it appears to disappear in special hospital populations that receive excellent health care. . . . [By contrast,] Children of older mothers are consistently less healthy at birth than children of average age mothers. This is likely to be a true biological effect" (Hofferth 1987:203). A similar relationship appears to hold for maternal mortality; that is, "increased age appears to be associated with increased rate of death" (Hofferth 1987:176). These findings strongly suggest that the adverse consequences of adolescent childbirth will be found unless "excellent health care" is provided. For a poor, adolescent, pregnant female that is anything but a sure thing. In this sense it is poverty, not age, that proves to be the problem. Indeed, in operational terms, age has become the proxy for poverty, as adolescent pregnancy programs have targeted the disadvantaged to the general exclusion of middle-class young people.

Finally, and ironically, a focus on the teenage years may well have the unintended effect of reducing the general public's sympathy and support for programs designed to help. This span of human development is one that all adults have experienced, but it is unlikely that many people who shape public policy have been mothers in their teens or the male partners of females who were. The teens at risk of early parenthood are apt to be regarded as "other people's kids," with all that phrase connotes regarding their perceived deviance and potential for unwelcome dependency. If this is so, focusing on *teen age* may have the perverse effect of serving to distance the average consumer of policy from the population selected for solicitous attention.

Nevertheless, with all the limitations just described, age remains useful in framing policy for this population.

Conclusion

Perhaps we should conclude that there are two teenage parenthood problems. One concerns school-age adolescents, the other females of eighteen and nineteen who account for most of the births to teenagers. Although these two populations of young mothers share the vulnerability associated with off-time parenthood, the differences between them suggest that parenthood will have a sufficiently dissimilar effect on their lives, in the short run and the long, to justify separate treatment under public policy.

For the school-age group, the advent of children threatens to interrupt schooling, diminish their freedom to test out new roles, and skew the defining of lifetime goals and priorities. School-age teens are, in our culture, at a pivotal point of development. The older group, by contrast, is farther advanced on the path to adulthood.

Legally these teens are adults, and socially, for the most part, they will have completed a major task of adolescence—schooling—and had the opportunity to experiment with adult roles, including work. Living an additional four years beyond one's fourteenth birthday, after all, represents a gain in experience of over 25 percent. For women of eighteen or nineteen, teenage parenthood is less an interruption of developmental assignments (although a moderated effect may still apply) than a diversion of time and energy from employment or further education and a potential threat of economic dependency and poverty. Moreover, while many pregnancy prevention programs have served a wide range of ages, from very young adolescents to adults under age twenty, the policy concerns that animate the public's interest appear to be quite distinct. For school-age teens, moral and prudential considerations seem to dominate, whereas among the eighteen- to nineteen-year-olds, with the exception of abortion, protection of the public fisc through reduction of welfare costs is the most widely discussed issue.

The differences between these groups should lead us to consider directing policy attention placed on teenage pregnancy and parenthood to females under eighteen. What reasons might justify this course of action? First of all, it seems obvious that a younger group is a better target for prevention. Of all the strategies for dealing with adolescent pregnancy and parenthood, preventing these occurrences works best. During the early teens, when curiosity and anxiety over personal sexual development run especially high, there is an opportunity to instruct adolescents about their sexuality and the considerations they should bring to bear on decisions relative to the onset of coitus. Clearly, this opportunity is shared with parents and peers, playing important if variable roles. From the standpoint of public policy, however, the early teens offer a propitious time to ensure that a certain level of information and understanding is possessed by all. Typically, such an objective translates into a responsibility for the schools, although churches and other voluntary associations will assuredly assert their prerogatives to shape adolescents' values.

Yet another reason for emphasizing pregnancy prevention among this population has to do with education. In the contemporary job market, individuals lacking high school diplomas are at a severe competitive disadvantage. Indeed, with the widespread lengthening of educational careers, many entrants into the labor force possess additional credentials. At minimum, however, completion of high school is necessary for entry into nearly all types of employment. Failure to pass this milestone is a serious obstacle to financial independence. School drop-outs who bear children should be particular targets of intervention because of their poor track record in completing high school (Upchurch and McMarthy 1990); this group and other young adolescents with school-based problems are of prime concern in pregnancy prevention programs focused on under-eighteen teenagers in order to forestall the damaging consequences that otherwise flow from failure to complete schooling. It is also worth noting that the long-range self-interest of the adolescent and society's stake in an educated citizenry are equally at risk; efforts to achieve either goal assist the other.

Priority attention to this group is further indicated by practical considerations. Nearly all young adolescents are in school. Thus, they are easy to identify and reach. In short, a plan for reaching out to younger adolescents intuitively promises greater preventive efficacy than later interventions because it should be possible at least to cushion the influence of misinformation and peer pressure. Exactly how to achieve these results, and indeed to what extent they can be obtained, is uncertain, given the shortage of carefully constructed evaluations. Notwithstanding, two considerations support this focus: encouraging evidence from anecdotal reports and the few evaluations conducted to date; and the generally positive influence of these programs on the lives of those adolescents served even where prevention, by any measure, has not been achieved.

Where, then, would a redirection of public policy leave older teenagers? Are they not also in need of the various services school-age adolescents receive? For many the answer is a resounding "yes," and in any event drawing a line by age inevitably imports an element of arbitrariness. Nevertheless, public policy should not give special attention to this age-group.

These men and women of eighteen or older are adults, with all that implies regarding choice and responsibility. They are, as well, free agents in the sense that they are no longer anchored in an institution of compulsory attendance, nor are they apt to be so firmly embedded in their families. Efforts by the state to control their personal decisions on matters related to sexual behavior would, in any event, be beyond the reach of the public policies this nation would accept. But what of their needs for the kinds of programmatic assistance and supports that have flourished in a number of communities?

There can be no doubt as to the unmet need that exists among the poor older adolescent population and, for that matter, among those in their early twenties, whose social and economic situation closely parallels older adolescents'. Health care, remedial education, job training and employment opportunity, and measures directed at reducing the structural conditions underlying individual disadvantage would make a big difference to millions of young adults. In short, what the preponderance of poor eighteen- and nineteen-year-old mothers (and fathers) require is a structure of support and opportunities similar to those which aid middle-class youth in the transition from dependency to semi-dependency to relative autonomy.

Such basic needs call for generalized response. Addressing them through pregnancy prevention programs is understandable, but in the long term the public interest is better served by attending to such widely required supports and services as matters of importance in their own right, not as the offspring of adolescent pregnancy initiatives. For reasons of equity and adequacy, that is the course policymaking should follow.

But what about welfare, one may ask? How should we think about its relationship to teen parenthood? What to do about the welfare problem is certainly beyond the scope of this work, but a few observations deserve recording. While international comparisons must be drawn with caution, it is worth noting that the rates of adolescent pregnancy and birth are much lower in industrialized countries with more generous welfare provisions than exist in the United States (Jones et al. 1986; Hoem this volume).

It is also important to remind ourselves that welfare benefits not only provide support for the mother; they do likewise for the child or children. And children are long-claimed subjects of a tradition of state beneficence in recognition of the public interest in future citizens' well-being. (The evolution of a number of adolescent pregnancy programs to include services to young parents and their children bespeaks the power of this public claim.) Nevertheless, certain recent developments seem to undercut this position. The current policy stance mandating young welfare mothers to work or participate in placement and training activities by implication undercuts the social priority attached to maternal care of children or else it renders the unspoken judgment that other caretakers are superior to the kids' own parents.

Additional welfare reform proposals are in circulation, including those to block what are currently automatic increases in AFDC benefit level following the birth of a child subsequent to the mother's initial enrolment in the program. If payment levels are maintained at the previous amount designated for a family of two or three, for example, it is assumed that the incentive to become pregnant and bear the child will be reduced. Several states have considered such legislation (Davis 1991). But how does the third or fourth member of the family derive support? The obvious answer, so far as AFDC cash assistance goes, is through spreading further the existing benefit dollars. Another idea that has been bruited about is requiring implantation of Norplant to prevent future conception among women whose child-rearing capabilities are sorely wanting (Cantwell 1991).

Perhaps most worrisome about proposals of this kind is the meanness of spirit surrounding their public display. This is not to say that the welfare "problem" is an illegitimate construct or that people may not differ sharply regarding its remediation. They may—and do (Piven and Cloward 1971; Murray 1984; Ellwood 1988). Evidence of mounting frustration gives rise to grave concern, however, when solutions proposed for "deviant" parenthood partake of Orwellian measures like forced use of Norplant to prevent future childbirths. Lionel Trilling's words of caution are apposite in this connection: "Some paradox of our nature leads us, when once we have made our fellow men [and women] the object of our enlightened interest, to go on to make them objects of our pity, then our wisdom, ultimately our coercion" (Trilling 1953:214).

Adolescent parenthood is off-time; it is risky for the mother and her child; it is costly for society. We have gained a better understanding of its risks and costs through recent experience and study and as a result should be better prepared to attack the future. Clearly poverty is the substratum on which most of these families are built. Their needs overall exceed the resources available to pregnancy prevention programs, but these have told us more about the nature of adolescents' needs and strategies to address them. For school-age adolescents, in particular, the merits of intervention have been put forward.

It can be predicted with assurance that adolescent pregnancy and paarenthood will not disappear; nor, unless trends change radically, will these events commonly occur within the shelter of marriage. Very few would voice dissent to promoting stable marriages as a goal, but this has proved over centuries to be an elusive goal of public policy, more amenable it appears to influence by parents, kin, churches, and the broad tides of sociopolitical and economic change. Most policymakers would like to find a good "solution"—and turn their attention to the next problem instead. But in the near future this is probably not to be. The task remains to guide young adolescents along the route to responsible self-regulation and to charge the larger society with demonstrating to adolescents that such a course is worth their while.

NOTES

This chapter has benefited from the comments of Andrew Boxer, Laurence Lynn, Dolores Norton and Franklin Zimring.

1. Katchadourian (1990) speculates about the difficulties parents have talking to their children on this subject: "It has become standard practice to berate American parents for their failure to educate their children about sexuality. But there is no evidence that parents in other comparable cultures do a significantly better job. Perhaps there are deeper reasons why it is hard to talk to one's own children about sex no matter how well-informed or enlightened a parent may be. Talking about sex is a form of sexual interaction, and its avoidance may be part of the incest taboo. The adolescence of children often coincides with the middle age of parents. Both are periods of transition, with their particular anxieties, including sexual concerns. To expect parents to tend personally to the sexual instruction of their children while they themselves are in search of answers in their own lives may be unrealistic" (343).

2. An observation on the phenomenon of sexual victimization should be noted. Clearly, some sexual relations involving adolescent girls (and boys as well) are not consensual in nature (Gershenson et al. 1989). Over 50 percent of the victims in indicated child sexual abuse cases in Illinois in fiscal year 1984 were between the ages of ten and eighteen, with the overwhelming proportion of victims (83%) being female (Testa and Lawlor 1985:78, table 41). Some of these cases reveal the vulnerability of children to their regular caretakers. Some—but how many, we cannot say—also result in pregnancies attributable to incest or rape. It does appear that concentrating on the problem of teenage premarital sexual relations diverts attention from the fact that on occasion these relations are anything but consensual. When the topic of child sexual abuse is on the table, this awareness is central; when, however, adolescent pregnancy is under consideration, it is apt to fade from view. We should remember that some adolescents—girls *and* boys—are sexual victims and that, of the females in this group, some will become pregnant as a result.

Bibliography

Abrahamse, A. F., P. A. Morrison, and L. T. Waite (1988). "Teenagers Willing to Consider Single Parenthood: Who Is at Greatest Risk?" *Family Planning Perspectives* 20:13–18.

Abukhanfusa, K. (1987). *Piskan och moroten: Om könens tilldelning av skydigheter och rättigheter i det svenska socialforsäkringssystemet 1913–1983.* Stockholm: Carlssons.

Alan Guttmacher Institute (AGI) (1976). *11 Million Teenagers: What Can Be Done about the Epidemic of Adolescent Pregnancies in the United States.* New York: Planned Parenthood Federation of America.

Alcott, W. A. (1856). *Physiology of Marriage.* Boston: John P. Jewett.

Allen, W. W. (1978). "The Search for Applicable Theories of Black Family Life." *Journal of Marriage and the Family* 40:117–129.

American Public Welfare Association (1986). *One Child in Four.* New York: APWA.

Anderson, E. (1989). "Sex Codes and Family Life among Poor Inner-City Youths." *Annals of the American Academy of Political and Social Science* 501:59–78.

——— (1990). *Streetwise: Race, Class, and Change in an Urban Community.* Chicago: University of Chicago Press.

Andrews, R. H., Jr., and A. H. Cohn (1977). "PINS Processing in New York: An Evaluation." In L. E. Teitelbaum and A. R. Gough (Eds.), *Beyond Control: Status Offenders in the Juvenile Court.* Cambridge, MA: Ballinger.

Aponte, R. (1988). "Conceptualizing the Underclass: An Alternative Perspective." Paper presented to annual meeting of the American Sociological Association, Atlanta, GA.

Ariès, P. (1962). *Centuries of Childhood.* Trans. R. Baldick, New York: Vintage.

Arvidsson, A., et al. (1982). *Kvinnor och barn: Intervjuer med kvinnor om familj och arbete.* Statistics Sweden, Stockholm: Information i prognosfrågor 1982:4.

Auletta, K. (1983). *The Underclass.* New York: Random House.

Baltes, P. B., H. W. Reese, and L. P. Lipsitt (1980). "Life-Span Developmental Psychology." *Annual Review of Psychology* 31:65–100.

Bane, M. J., and P. A. Jargowsky (1988). "The Links between Government Policy and Family Structure: What Matters and What Doesn't." In A. J. Cherlin (Ed.), *The Changing American Family and Public Policy.* Washington, D.C.: Urban Institute.

Banfield, E. C. (1974). *The Unheavenly City Revisited.* Boston: Little, Brown and Co.

Bell, W. (1965). *Aid to Dependent Children.* New York: Columbia University Press.

Belle, D. (1982). "Social Ties and Social Support." In D. Belle (Ed.), *Lives in Stress: Women and Depression.* Beverly Hills, CA.: Sage.

Berg, B. J. (1978). *The Remembered Gate: The Origins of American Feminism: The Woman and the City, 1800–1860.* New York: Oxford University Press.

Bernhardt, E. (1988). "The Choice of Part-Time Work among Swedish One-Child Mothers." *European Journal of Population* 4:117–144.

Bernhardt, E., and B. Hoem (1986). "Cohabitation and Social Background: Trends Observed for Swedish Women Born 1936–60." *European Journal of Population* 1:375–395.

Berzonsky, M. D. (1978). "Formal Reasoning in Adolescence: An Alternative View." *Adolescence* 13:279–290.

Besharov, D. (1989). "Targeting Long-Term Welfare Recipients." In P. Cottingham and D. Ellwood (Eds.), *Welfare Policy for the 1990s.* Cambridge, MA: Harvard University Press.

Billingsley, A. (1968). *Black Families in White America.* Englewood Cliffs, NJ: Prentice-Hall.

Billy, J.O.G., and J. R. Udry (1985). "Patterns of Adolescent Friendship and Effects on Sexual Behavior." *Social Psychology Quarterly* 48:27–41.

Bjerén, G. (1981). "Female and Male in a Swedish Forest Region: Old Roles under New Conditions." *Antropoloqiska Studier* 30/31:56–85.

Blassingame, J. W. (1979). *The Slave Community: Plantation Life in the Antebellum South.* New York: Oxford University Press.

Blos, P. (1962). *On Adolescence: A Psychoanalytic Interpretation.* New York: Free Press.

Bolton, F. G., Jr. (1980). *The Pregnant Adolescent: Problems of Premature Parenthood.* Beverly Hills, CA: Sage.

Boxer, A. M., R. A. Levinson, and A. C. Petersen (1989). "Adolescent Sexuality." In J. Worrell and F. Danner (Eds.), *The Adolescent as Decision-Maker.* New York: Academic Press.

Breslow, N., J. Lubin, P. Marek, and B. Langholz (1983). "Multiplicative Models and Cohort Analysis." *Journal of the American Statistical Association* 78:1–12.

Brodkin, E. Z. (1990). "Implementation as Policy Politics." In D. Calista and D. Palumbo (Eds.), *Implementation and Public Policy: Opening the Black Box.* Westport, CT: Greenwood.

Brodkin, E. Z., and R. Shaikh (1986). "Anatomy of a Chemical Crisis." In F. Homberger (Ed.), *Safety and Evaluation of Chemicals.* Basel: Karger.

Brooks-Gunn, J., C. Boyer, and K. Hein (1988). "Preventing HIV Infection and AIDS in Children and Adolescents." *American Psychologist* 43:958–964.

Brooks-Gunn, J., and P. Chase-Lansdale (1991). "Children Having Children:

Effects on the Family System." *Pediatric Annals* 20:467, 470–471, 473–474, 476, 478, 480–481.

Brooks-Gunn, J., and F. F. Furstenberg, Jr. (1989). "Adolescent Sexual Behavior." *American Psychologist* 44:249–257.

Brown, L. K., G. K. Fritz, and V. J. Barone (1989). "The Impact of AIDS Education on Junior and Senior High School Students." *Journal of Adolescent Health Care* 10:386–392.

Brumberg, J. J. (1985). " 'Ruined' Girls: Changing Community Responses to Illegitimacy in Upstate New York, 1890–1930." *Journal of Social History* 18:363–374.

Brunswick, A. F., and A. A. Aidala (1991). "Adult Consequences of Adolescent Childbearing: The Longitudinal Harlem Health Study." In R. L. Taylor (Ed.), *Black Youth: Perspectives on Their Social and Economic Status.* Newbury Park, CA: Sage.

Buchmann, M. (1989). *The Script of Life in Modern Society: Entry into Adulthood in a Changing World.* Chicago: University of Chicago Press.

Bumpass, L., and J. A. Sweet (1972). "Differentials in Marital Stability: 1970." *American Sociological Review* 37:754–766.

Burgess, E. W. (1926). "The Family as a Unit of Interacting Personalities." *Family* 7:3–9.

——— (1939). Introduction to *The Negro Family in the United States,* by E. F. Frazier. Chicago: University of Chicago Press.

Burton, L. M. (1990). "Teenage Childbearing as an Alternative Life-Course Strategy in Multigenerational Black Families." *Human Nature* 1:123–143.

Burton, L. M., and V. L. Bengtson (1985). "Black Grandmothers; Issues of Timing and Continuity of Roles." In V. L. Bengtson and J. F. Robertson (Eds.), *Grandparenthood.* Beverly Hills, CA: Sage.

Butler, J. R. (1988). "Rethinking Teenage Childbearing: Is Sexual Abuse a Missing Link?" Unpublished master's thesis. Pennsylvania State University, University Park.

Calhoun, A. (1960). *A Social History of the American Family.* 3 vols. New York: Barnes and Noble.

Calleman, C., L. Lagercrantz, and K. Widerberg (1984). *Kvinnoreformer pa mannens villkor.* Lund: Studentlitteratur.

Campbell, A. A. (1968). "The Role of Family Planning in the Reduction of Poverty." *Journal of Marriage and the Family* 30:236–245.

Cantwell, M. (1991). "Coercion and Contraception." *New York Times,* January 27, Sec. 4, p. 16.

Caplan, G. (1964). *Principles of Preventive Psychiatry.* New York: Basic Books.

Card, J. J., and L. Wise (1978). "Teenage Mothers and Teenage Fathers: The Impact of Early Childbearing on the Parents' Personal and Professional Lives." *Family Planning Perspectives* 10:199–205.

Center for the Study of Social Policy (1984). "The 'Flip Side' of Black Families Headed by Women: The Economic Status of Black Men." Working paper. Washington, D.C.

Centers for Disease Control (1989). "AIDS and Human Immunodeficiency Virus Infection in the U.S.: 1988 update." *Morbidity and Mortality Weekly Report 38* (No. S-4), May 12. Washington: GPO.

────── (1990). "HIV-Related Knowledge and Behaviors among High School Students—Selected U.S. Sites, 1989." *Morbidity and Mortality Weekly Report 39* (No. 23), June 15. Washington: GPO.

────── (1991). "Premarital Sexual Experience among Adolescent Women—United States, 1970–1988." *Morbidity and Mortality Weekly Report 39* (Nos. 51, 52), January 4. Washington: GPO.

Chambers, D. L. (1979). *Making Fathers Pay: The Enforcement of Child Support*. Chicago: University of Chicago Press.

Chase-Lansdale, P. L., and J. Brooks-Gunn (1991). "Research and Programs." *Family Relations* 40:396–404.

Chase-Lansdale, P. L., and M. A. Vinovskis (1987). "Should We Discourage Teenage Marriage?" *Public Interest* 87:23–37.

Cherlin, A. J. (1992). *Marriage, Divorce and Remarriage*. Cambridge: Harvard University Press.

Children's Defense Fund (1987a). *Adolescent Pregnancy: An Anatomy of a Social Problem in Search of Comprehensive Solutions*. Washington, DC: Children's Defense Fund.

────── (1987b). *Declining Earnings of Young Men: Their Relation to Poverty, Teen Pregnancy, and Family Formation*. Washington, DC: Children's Defense Fund.

────── (1988). *Teenage Pregnancy: An Advocate's Guide to the Numbers*. Washington, DC: Children's Defense Fund.

────── (1989). *A Children's Defense Budget*. Washington, DC: Children's Defense Fund.

────── (1990). *SOS America: A Children's Defense Budget*. Washington, DC: Children's Defense Fund.

Chilman, C. S. (1978). *Adolescent Sexuality in a Changing American Society: Social and Psychosocial Perspectives*. Washington: GPO, DHEW Publication No. (NIH) 79-1426.

────── (1983). *Adolescent Sexuality in a Changing American Society*. New York: Wiley.

────── (1986). "Some Psychosocial Aspects of Adolescent Sexual and Contraceptive Behaviors in a Changing American Society." In J. B. Lancaster and B. A. Hamburg (Eds.), *School-Age Pregnancy and Parenthood: Biosocial Dimensions*. New York: Aldine de Gruyter.

Clark, K. B. (1967). *Dark Ghetto: Dilemmas of Social Power*. New York: Harper Torchbooks.

Clark, S. D., L. S. Zabin, and J. B. Hardy (1984). "Sex, Contraception, and Parenthood: Experience and Attitudes among Urban Black Young Men." *Family Planning Perspectives* 16:77–82.

Cobb, R. W., and C. D. Elder (1975). *Participation in American Politics*. Baltimore: Johns Hopkins University Press.

Cohen, R. S., B. J. Cohler, and S. H. Weissman (1984). *Parenthood: A Psycho-Dynamic Perspective*. New York: Guilford.

Cohler, B. J. (in press). "Becoming Adolescent Parents: Strain in Off-Time Transition to Parenthood." In A. L. Greene and A. M. Boxer (Eds.), *Adolescence and Life-Course Transitions*. Hillsdale, NJ: L. Erlbaum.

Coleman, J. (1961). *The Adolescent Society: The Social Life of the Teenager and Its Impact on Education*. Glencoe, IL: Free Press.

Colletta, N. D. (1983). "At Risk of Depression: A Study of Young Mothers." *Journal of Genetic Psychology* 142:301–310.

Committee for Economic Development (1987). *Children in Need: Investment Strategies For the Educationally Disadvantaged.* New York: CED.

Congressional Budget Office (1982). *Improving Youth Employment Prospects: Issues and Options.* Washington: Congress of the United States.

———— (1990). *Sources of Support for Adolescent Mothers.* Washington: Congress of the United States.

Constanzo, P. R., and M. E. Shaw (1966). "Conformity as a Function of Age Level." *Child Development* 37:967–975.

Corbett, T., J. Deloya, W. Manning, and L. Uhr (1989). "Learnfare: The Wisconsin Experience." *Focus* 12:1–10.

Cremin, L. A. (1980). *American Education: The National Experience, 1783–1876.* New York: Harper & Row.

Crenson, Matthew A. (1971). *The Unpolitics of Air Pollution.* Baltimore: Johns Hopkins University Press.

Crockett, L. J., L. Dorn, and A. C. Petersen (1990). "Cross-Sex Interaction in Early Adolescence: Effects of Pubertal Maturation." Unpublished manuscript.

Crockett, L. J., and A. C. Petersen. (1987). "Pubertal Status and Psychosocial Development: Findings from the Early Adolescence Study." In R. M. Lerner and T. T. Foch (Eds.), *Biological and Psychosocial Interactions in Early Adolescence.* Hillsdale, NJ: Lawrence Erlbaum.

Danzig, R., and P. Szanton (1986). *National Service: What Would It Mean?* Lexington, MA: Lexington Books.

Danziger, S. H., and D. H. Weinberg (Eds.) (1986). *Fighting Poverty: What Works and What Doesn't.* Cambridge, MA: Harvard University Press.

Darabi, K. F., S. Gustavus, and A. Rosenfield (1979). "A Perspective on Adolescent Fertility in Developing Countries." *Studies in Family Planning* 10:300–303.

Darity, W., Jr., and S. L. Myers, Jr. (1984). "Does Welfare Dependency Cause Female Headship? The Case of the Black Family." *Journal of Marriage and the Family* 46: 224–235.

Dash, L. (1989). *When Children Want Children: The Urban Crisis of Teenage Childbearing.* New York: Morrow.

Davis, A., B. B. Gardner, and M. R. Gardner (1941). *Deep South: A Social Anthropological Study of Caste and Class.* Chicago: University of Chicago Press.

Davis, K., M. Bernstam, and R. Ricardo-Campbell (Eds.) (1986). *Below Replacement Fertility in Industrial Societies: Causes, Consequences, Policies.* Suppl. to *Population and Development Review,* vol. 12.

Davis, M. F. (1991). "War on Poverty, War on Women." *New York Times,* August 3, Sec. A, p. 19.

Degler, C. N. (1980). *At Odds: Women and the Family in America from the Revolution to the Present.* New York: Oxford University Press.

Dembo, R. (1988). "Delinquency among Black Male Youth." In J. T. Gibbs (Ed.), *Young, Black and Male in America: An Endangered Species.* Dover, MA: Auburn House.

Demos, J. (1970). *A Little Commonwealth: Family Life in Plymouth Colony.* New York: Oxford University Press.

Demos, J., and V. Demos (1969). "Adolescence in Historical Perspective." *Journal of Marriage and the Family* 31:632–638.

Dienes, C. T. (1972). *Law, Politics and Birth Control.* Urbana: University of Illinois Press.

Dollard, J. (1937). *Caste and Class in a Southern Town*. New Haven, CT: Yale University Press.

Donovan, J. E., and R. Jessor (1985). "Structure of Problem Behavior in Adolescence and Young Adulthood." *Journal of Consulting and Clinical Psychology* 53:890–904.

Downs, A. (1972). "Up and Down with Ecology—'The Issue Attention Cycle.' " *Public Interest* 32:38–50.

Drake, St. C., and H. Cayton (1945). *Black Metropolis: A Study of Negro Life in a Northern City,* vol. 2. New York: Harcourt, Brace.

Dryfoos, J. (1988). *Putting the Boys in the Picture: A Review of Programs to Promote Sexual Responsibility among Young Males*. Santa Cruz, CA: Network Publications.

——— (1990). *Adolescents at Risk: Prevalence and Prevention*. New York: Oxford University Press.

Duncan, G. J., M. Hill, and S. D. Hoffman (1988). "Welfare Dependence Within and Across Generations." *Science* 239:467.

Duncan, G. J., and S. D. Hoffman (1988). "The Use and Effects of Welfare: A Survey of Recent Evidence." *Social Service Review* 62:238–257.

——— (1991). "Teenage Underclass Behavior and Subsequent Poverty: Have the Rules Changed?" In C. Jencks and P. E. Peterson (Eds.), *The Urban Underclass*. Washington, D.C.: Brookings Institution.

Durch, J. S. (1980). *Nuptiality Patterns in Developing Countries: Implications for Fertility*. Washington, D.C.: Population Reference Bureau, No. 30.

Earle, A. M. (1895). *Colonial Dames and Goodwives*. Boston: Macmillan.

Eberly, D., and M. Sherraden. (1990). *The Moral Equivalent of War? A Study of Non-Military Service in Nine Nations*. New York, Westport, CT, and London: Greenwood.

Edelman, M. W. (1987). *Families in Peril: An Agenda for Social Change*. Cambridge, MA: Harvard University Press.

Edwards, L., M. Steinman, K. Arnold, and E. Hakanson (1980). "Adolescent Pregnancy Prevention Services in High School Clinics." *Family Planning Perspectives* 12:6–14.

Egeland, B., D. Jacobvitz, and L. A. Sroufe. (1988). "Breaking the Cycle of Abuse." *Child Development* 59:1080–1088.

Elder, G. H., Jr. (1975). "Age Differentiation and the Life Course." *Annual Review of Sociology* 1:165–190.

——— (1985). "Perspectives on the Life Course." In G. H. Elder, Jr., *Life Course Dynamics: Trajectories and Transitions, 1968–1988*. Ithaca: Cornell University Press.

Elkind, D. (1981). *Children and Adolescents: Interpretive Essays on Je* 3d ed. New York: Oxford University Press.

Elliott, D. S. (in press). "Health Enhancing and Health Compromi styles." In S. Millstein, A. C. Petersen, and E. O. Nightingale (Eds.), *cent Health Promotion*. New York: Oxford University Press.

Ellwood, D. T. (1986). "Targeting 'Would Be' Long Term Recipients of AFDC Princeton, NJ: Mathematica Policy Research.

——— (1988). *Poor Support: Poverty in the American Family*. New York: Basic Books.

——— (1990). "Men and Marriage in the Black Community." *Research Bulle-*

tin, Fall, Malcolm Wiener Center for Social Policy, John F. Kennedy School of Government, Harvard University, Cambridge, MA.

Ellwood, D. T., and M. J. Bane (1984). *The Impact of AFDC on Family Structure and Living Arrangements.* Report for U.S. Department of Health and Human Services, Grant 92A-82. Mimeo. John F. Kennedy School of Government, Harvard University, Cambridge, MA.

Engerman, S. I. (1977). "Black Fertility and Family Structure in the U.S., 1880–1940." *Journal of Family History* 6:117–138.

Ensminger, M. E. (1987). "Adolescent Sexual Behavior as It Relates to Other Transition Behaviors in Youth." In S. L. Hofferth and C. D. Hayes (Eds.), *Risking the Future: Adolescent Sexuality, Pregnancy, and Childbearing,* vol. 2. Washington: National Academy Press.

Etzler, C. (1988). "Första barnet, en demografisk studie av barnafödandet bland svenska kvinnor födda 1936–60." *Stockholm Research Reports in Demography,* No. 44.

Eveleth, P. B. (1986). "Timing of Menarche: Secular Trend and Population Differences." In J. Lancaster and B. Hamburg (Eds.), *School-Age Pregnancy and Parenthood: Biosocial Dimensions.* New York: Aldine de Gruyter.

Fallers, L. A. (1973). *Inequality: Social Stratification Reconsidered.* Chicago: University of Chicago Press.

Farber, N. (1987). "Antecedents to Unmarried Adolescent Motherhood: A Cross-Class and Cross-Racial Analysis." Ph.D. diss., School of Social Service Administration, University of Chicago.

Featherman, D. L., and R. M. Hauser (1978). *Opportunity and Change.* New York: Academic Press.

Fine, M. (1988). "Sexuality, Schooling, and Adolescent Females: The Missing Discourse of Desire." *Harvard Educational Review* 58:29–53.

Fisher, W. A., D. Byrne, M. Edmunds, C. T. Miller, K. Kelley, and L. A. White (1979). "Psychological and Situation-Specific Correlates of Contraceptive Behavior among University Women." *Journal of Sex Research* 15:38–55.

Fogel, R. (1986). "Nutrition and the Decline in Mortality since 1700: Some Additional Preliminary Findings." Working Paper Series, no. 1802, National Bureau of Economic Research, Cambridge, MA.

Forneng, S. (1987). *Från skola till arbetsmarknad. Tendenser på ungdomarnas ʼtsmarknad.* Stockholm: Statistics Sweden, Information om arbetsmark-ʼ, 2.

J. D., and S. Singh (1990). "The Sexual and Reproductive Behavior of ʼan Women, 1982–1988." *Family Planning Perspectives* 22:206–214.

(1981). "The Family's Role in Adolescent Sexual Behavior." In T. ːd.), *Teenage Pregnancy in a Family Context: Implications for Policy.* ⏑lphia: Temple University Press.

⏑, D. L. (1988*a*). "The Impact of Early Childbearing on Developmental ⏑utcomes: The Case of Black Adolescent Parenting." *Family Relations* 37:268–274.

——— (1988*b*). "Race, Class and Adolescent Pregnancy: An Ecological Analysis." *American Journal of Orthopsychiatry* 58:339–354.

Frazier, E. F. (1938). "Some Effects of the Depression on the Negro in Northern Cities." *Science and Society* 2:495–496.

———— (1966). *The Negro Family in the United States,* rev. ed. Chicago: University of Chicago Press.

Freeman, R. B., and H. Holzer (1986). *The Black Youth Employment Crisis.* Chicago: University of Chicago Press.

Frisch, R. E., and J. W. McArthur (1974). "Menstrual Cycles: Fatness as a Determinant of Minimum Weight Necessary for Their Maintenance or Onset." *Science* 435:949–951.

Furstenberg, F. F., Jr. (1976). *Unplanned Parenthood: The Social Consequences of Teenage Childbearing.* New York: Free Press.

———— (1988). "Bringing Back the Shotgun Wedding." *Public Interest* 90: 121–127.

———— (1990). "Coming of Age in a Changing Family System." In S. S. Feldman and G. R. Elliott (Eds.), *At the Threshold: The Developing Adolescent.* Cambridge, MA: Harvard University Press.

———— (in press). "How Families Manage Risk and Opportunity in Dangerous Neighborhoods." In W. J. Wilson (Ed.), *Sociology and the Public Agenda.* Beverly Hills, CA: Sage Publications.

Furstenberg, F. F., Jr., and J. Brooks-Gunn (1986). "Teenage Childbearing: Causes, Consequences, and Remedies." In L. H. Aiken and D. Mechanic (Eds.), *Applications of Social Science to Clinical Medicine and Health Policy.* New Brunswick, NJ: Rutgers University Press.

Furstenberg, F. F., Jr., J. Brooks-Gunn, and L. Chase-Lansdale (1989). "Teenage Pregnancy and Childbearing." *American Psychologist* 44:313–320.

Furstenberg, F. F., Jr., J. Brooks-Gunn, and S. P. Morgan (1987). *Adolescent Mothers in Later Life.* Cambridge: Cambridge University Press.

Furstenberg, F. F., Jr., and A. Crawford (1978). "Family Support: Helping Teenage Mothers to Cope." *Family Planning Perspectives* 10:322–333.

Furstenberg, F. F., Jr., and K. M. Harris (1990). "The Disappearing American Father? Divorce and the Waning Significance of Biological Parenthood." Paper presented at the Albany Conference on Demographic Perspectives on the American Family: Patterns and Prospects.

Furstenberg, F. F., Jr., R. Lincoln, and J. Menken (1981). *Teenage Sexuality, Pregnancy and Childbearing.* Philadelphia: University of Pennsylvania Press.

Furstenberg, F. F., Jr., K. A. Moore, and J. L. Peterson (1986). "Sex Education and Sexual Experience among Adolescents." *American Journal of Public Health* 75:1221–1222.

Gagnon, J. (1989). "Sexuality across the Life Course in the United States." In C. F. Turner, H. G. Miller, and L. E. Moses (Eds.), *AIDS: Sexual Behavior and Intravenous Drug Use.* Washington: National Academy Press.

Gamson, J. (1990). "Rubber Wars: Struggles over the Condom in the United States." *Journal of the History of Sexuality* 1:262–282.

Gamson, W. A. (1975). *The Strategy of Social Protest.* Homewood, IL: Dorsey.

Gans, H. (1990). "Deconstructing the Underclass: The Term's Danger as a Planning Concept." *Journal of the American Planning Association* 56: 271–349.

Garfinkel, I., and S. McLanahan (1985). "The Feminization of Poverty: Nature, Causes and a Partial Cure." Institute for Research on Poverty Discussion Papers, University of Wisconsin–Madison.

———— (1986). *Single Mothers and Their Children: A New American Dilemma.* Washington, DC: Urban Institute Press.

Garmezy, N., and M. Rutter (1983). *Stress, Coping and Development in Children.* New York: McGraw-Hill.

Gatlin, R. (1987). *American Women since 1945.* Jackson: University Press of Mississippi.

Genovese, E. D. (1974). *Roll, Jordan, Roll: The World the Slaves Made.* New York: Random House.

Geronimus, A. T. (1987). "On Teenage Childbearing and Neonatal Mortality in the United States." *Population and Development Review* 13:245–279.

———. (1991). "Teenage Childbearing and Social and Reproductive Disadvantage: The Evolution of Complex Questions and the Demise of Simple Answers." *Family Relations* 40:453–471.

Geronimus, A. T., and S. Korenman (1991). "The Social Consequences of Teen Childbearing Reconsidered." Working Paper No. 3701. Cambridge, MA: National Bureau of Economic Research.

Gershenson, H. P., J. S. Musick, H. S. Ruch-Ross, V. Magee, K. K. Rubino, and D. Rosenberg (1989). "The Prevalence of Coercive Sexual Experience among Teenage Mothers." *Journal of Interpersonal Violence* 4:204–219.

Gibbs, J. T. (1986). "Psychosocial Correlates of Sexual Attitudes and Behaviors in Urban Early Adolescent Females: Implications for Intervention." *Journal of Social Work and Human Sexuality* 5:81–97.

——— (1988*a*). "Conceptual, Methodological, and Sociocultural Issues in Black Youth Suicide: Implications for Assessment and Early Intervention." *Suicide and Life-Threatening Behavior* 18:73–87.

——— (Ed.) (1988*b*). *Young, Black and Male in America: An Endangered Species.* Dover, MA: Auburn House.

Gittler, J., M. Quigley-Rick, and M. J. Saks (1990). "Adolescent Health Care Decision Making: The Law and Public Policy." Working paper, Carnegie Council on Adolescent Development, Washington, D.C.

Glasgow, D. (1981). *The Black Underclass.* New York: Vintage.

Glazer, N., and D. P. Moynihan (1963). *Beyond the Melting Pot.* Cambridge, MA: MIT Press.

Glendon, M. A. (1981). *The New Family and the New Property.* Toronto: Butterworths.

——— (1989). *The Transformation of Family Law: State, Law, and Family in the United States and Western Europe.* Chicago and London: University of Chicago Press.

——— (1991). *Rights Talk.* New York: Free Press.

Greenberger, E., and L. Steinberg (1986). *When Teenagers Work: The Psychological and Social Costs of Adolescent Employment.* New York: Basic Books.

Greene, A. L., and A. M. Boxer (1986). "Daughters and Sons as Young Adults: Restructuring the Ties That Bind." In N. Datan, A. L. Greene, and H. W. Reese (Eds.), *Life-Span Developmental Psychology: Intergenerational Relations.* Hillsdale, NJ: L. Erlbaum.

Greven, P. J., Jr. (1970). *Four Generations: Population, Land, and Family in Colonial Andover, Massachusetts.* Ithaca, NY: Cornell University Press.

Griswold, R. L. (1982). *Family and Divorce in California, 1850–1900: Victorian Illusions and Everyday Realities.* Albany: State University of New York.

Grønbjerg, K., D. Street, and G. D. Suttles (1978). *Poverty and Social Change.* Chicago: University of Chicago Press.

Gross, J. (1988). "New York's Poorest Women Offered More AIDS Services." *New York Times,* March 6, p. 1.

Grossman, J. R. (1989). *Land of Hope: Chicago, Black Southerners, and the Great Migration.* Chicago and London: University of Chicago Press.

Gueron, J. M. (1990). "Work and Welfare: Lessons on Employment Programs." *Journal of Economic Perspectives* 4:79–98.

Gustafsson, S., and P. Lantz (1985). *Arbete och löner: Ekonomiska teorier och fakta kring skillnader mellan kvinnor och män.* Stockholm: Industriens utredningsintitut och Arbetslivscentrum.

Gutman, H. G. (1976). *The Black Family in Slavery and Freedom, 1750–1925.* New York: Pantheon.

Hamburg, B. A. (1986). "Subsets of Adolescent Mothers: Developmental, Biomedical, and Psychosocial Issues." In J. Lancaster and B. Hamburg (Eds.), *School-Age Pregnancy and Parenthood: Biosocial Dimensions.* New York: Aldine de Gruyter.

——— (1990). "Life Skills Training: Preventive Interventions for Young Adolescents." Report of the Life Skills Training Working Group, Carnegie Council on Adolescent Development, Washington, D.C.

Handler, J. F. (1987–1988). "The Transformation of Aid to Families with Dependent Children: The Family Support Act in Historical Context." *New York University Review of Law and Social Change* 16:457–523.

Handler, J. F., and Hasenfeld, Y. (1991). *The Moral Construction of Poverty: Welfare Reform in America.* Newbury Park, CA: Sage.

Harrington, M. (1962). *The Other America: Poverty in the United States.* New York: Macmillan.

Hayes, C. D. (Ed.) (1987). *Risking the Future: Adolescent Sexuality, Pregnancy, and Childbearing,* vol. 1. Washington: National Academy Press.

Heclo, H. (1978). "Issue Networks and the Executive Establishment." In A. King (Ed.), *The New American Political System.* Washington, DC: American Enterprise Institute.

Hein, K. (1989). "AIDS in Adolescence: Exploring the Challenge." *Journal of Adolescent Health Care* 10:10S–35S.

Heiss, J. (1972). "On the Transmission of Marital Instability in Black Families." *American Sociological Review* 37:82–92.

Henshaw, S. K., A. M. Kenney, D. Somberg, and J. Van Vort (1989). *Teenage Pregnancy in the United States: The Scope of the Problem and State Responses.* New York: Alan Guttmacher Institute.

Henshaw, S. K., L. M. Koonin, and J. C. Smith (1991). "Characteristics of U.S. Women Having Abortions, 1987." *Family Planning Perspectives* 23:75–81.

Herdt, G., and A. M. Boxer (1991). "Ethnographic Issues in the Study of AIDS." *Journal of Sex Research* 28:171–187.

Hetherington, E. M., K. A. Camara, and D. L. Featherman (1983). "Achievement and Intellectual Functioning of Children in One-Parent Households." In J. Spence (Ed.), *Achievement and Achievement Motivation.* San Francisco: W. H. Freeman.

Hilgartner, S., and C. L. Bosk (1988). "The Rise and Fall of Social Problems: A Public Arenas Model." *American Journal of Sociology* 94:53–78.

Hill, M., S. Augustiniak, and M. Ponza (1985). "The Impact of Parental Marital

Disruption on the Socioeconomic Attainment of Children as Adults." Unpublished paper, University of Michigan, Institute for Social Research, Ann Arbor.

Hilts, P. J. (1990). "Birth-Control Backlash." *New York Times Magazine,* 16 December, pp. 41, 55, 70, 72, 74.

Hindus, M. A., and D. S. Smith (1975). "Premarital Pregnancy in America 1640–1971." *Journal of Interdisciplinary History* 5:537–570.

Hingson, R., L. Strunin, and B. Berlin (1990). "Acquired Immunodeficiency Syndrome Transmission: Changes in Knowledge and Behaviors among Teenagers." *Pediatrics* 85:24–29.

Hoem, B. (1984). "Regional utveckling i det moderna samboendet, analysmetoder och resultat." *Stockholm Research Reports in Demography,* No. 22.

Hoem, B., and J. Hoem (1987). "Patterns of Deferment of First Births in Modern Sweden." *Stockholm Research Reports in Demography,* No. 42.

——. (1992). "The Disruption of Marital and Nonmarital Unions in Contemporary Sweden." In J. Trussell, R. Hankinson, and J. Tilton (Eds.), *Demographic Applications of Event History Analysis.* Oxford: Oxford University Press for the International Union of the Scientific Study of Population.

Hoem, J. (1985). "The Impact of Education on Modern Family-Union Initiation." *Stockholm Research Reports in Demography,* No. 27.

—— (1986). "The Impact of Education on Modern Family-Union Initiation." *European Journal of Population* 2:113–133. (Shorter version.)

Hoem, J., B. Rennermalm, and R. Selmer. (1990). "Restriction Biases in the Analysis of Births and Marriages to Cohabiting Women from Data on the Most Recent Conjugal Union Only." In K. U. Mayer and N. B. Tuma (Eds.), *Event History Analysis in Life Course Analysis.* Madison, WI: University of Wisconsin Press.

Hofferth, S. L. (1987). "The Children of Teen Childbearers." In S. L. Hofferth and C. D. Hayes (Eds.), *Risking the Future: Adolescent Sexuality, Pregnancy, and Childbearing,* vol. 2. Washington: National Academy Press.

—— (1991). "Programs for High Risk Adolescents: What Works?" *Evaluation and Program Planning* 14:3–16.

Hofferth, S. L., and C. D. Hayes (Eds.) (1987). *Risking the Future: Adolescent Sexuality, Pregnancy, and Childbearing,* vol. 2. Washington: National Academy Press.

Hofferth, S. L., and K. A. Moore (1979). "Early Childbearing and Later Economic Well-Being." *American Sociological Review* 44:784–815.

Hoffman, S., and J. Holmes (1976). "Husbands, Wives and Divorce." In J. N. Morgan (Ed.), *Five Thousand American Families: Patterns of Economic Progress.* Vol. 4. Ann Arbor: Institute for Social Research, University of Michigan Press.

Hogan, D. P. (1982a). "Adolescent Expectations about the Sequencing of Early Life Transitions." Unpublished manuscript, The University of Chicago.

——. (1982b). "Subgroup Variations in Early Life Transitions." In M. W. Riley, R. P. Abeles, and M. S. Teitelbaum (Eds.), *Aging from Birth to Death, Volume II: Sociotemporal Perspectives.* Boulder, CO: Westview.

—— (1984). "Structural and Normative Factors in Single Parenthood among Black Adolescents." Paper presented at the 1984 meeting of the American Sociological Association, San Antonio, TX.

Hogan, D. P., and N. M. Astone (1986). "The Transition to Adulthood." *Annual Review of Sociology* 12:109–130.

Hogan, D. P., and E. M. Kitagawa (1985). "The Impact of Social Status, Family Structure, and Neighborhood on the Fertility of Black Adolescents." *American Journal of Sociology* 90:825–855.

Hopkins, K. R. (1987). *Welfare Dependency: Behavior, Culture, and Public Policy.* Alexandria, VA: Hudson Institute.

Hwang, C. P., G. Elden, and C. Fransson (1984). "Arbetsgivares och arbetskamraters attityder till pappaledighet." Report No. 1, Psykologiska Institutionen, Goteborgs Universitet.

Illinois Caucus on Teenage Pregnancy (1986). "Homeless in Chicago: The Special Case of Pregnant and Parenting Teens." Chicago: Illinois Caucus on Teenage Pregnancy.

Ingram, M. (1987). *Church Courts, Sex and Marriage in England, 1570–1640.* Cambridge: Cambridge University Press.

Institute of Judicial Administration—American Bar Association, Juvenile Justice Standards Project (1977). *Standards Relating to Noncriminal Misbehavior.* Tentative draft. Cambridge, MA: Ballinger.

Jackson, J., and M. A. Vinovskis (1983). "Public Opinion, Elections, and the 'Single-Issue.' " In G. Y. Steiner (Ed.), *The Abortion Dispute and the American System.* Washington, DC: Brookings Institution.

Jackson, S. R. (1989). "Learnfare: The State's Perspective." *Focus* 12:11–14.

Janis, I. L., and L. Mann (1977). *Decision Making: A Psychological Analysis of Conflict, Choice and Commitment.* New York: Free Press.

Janowitz, M. (1983). *The Reconstruction of Patriotism: Education for Civic Consciousness.* Chicago and London: University of Chicago Press.

Jaynes, G. D., and R. M. Williams, Jr. (Eds.) (1989). *A Common Destiny: Blacks and American Society.* Washington: National Academy Press.

Jencks, C. (1989). "Which Underclass Is Growing? Recent Changes in Joblessness, Educational Attainment, Crime, Family Structure, and Welfare Dependency." Prepared for a conference on William Julius Wilson's *The Truly Disadvantaged,* sponsored by the Social Science Research Council and Northwestern University's Center for Urban Affairs and Policy Research, Evanston, IL.

Jessor, R., and S. L. Jessor (1977). *Problem Behavior and Psychosocial Development: A Longitudinal Study of Youth.* New York: Academic Press.

Jessor, S., and R. Jessor (1975). "Transition from Virginity to Nonvirginity among Youth: A Social-Psychological Study over Time." *Developmental Psychology* 11:473–484.

Johnson, B. (1978). "Women Who Head Families, 1970–1977: Their Numbers Rose, Incomes Lagged." *Monthly Labor Review* 101:32–37.

Johnson, C. S. (1934). *Shadow of the Plantation.* Chicago: University of Chicago Press.

Johnson, D. M., and R. Campbell (1981). *Black Migration in America: A Social Demographic History.* Durham, NC: Duke University Press.

Johnston, L. D., P. M. O'Malley, and J. F. Bachman (1987). *National Trends in Drug Use and Related Factors among American High School Students and Young Adults, 1975–1986.* Washington: National Institute of Drug Abuse.

Jones, A. H. (1980). *Wealth of a Nation to Be: The American Colonies on the Eve of the Revolution.* New York: Columbia University Press.

Jones, E. F., J. D. Forrest, N. Goldman, S. K. Henshaw, R. Lincoln, J. I. Rosoff, C. F. Westoff, and D. Wulf (1985). "Teenage Pregnancy in Developed

Countries: Determinants and Policy Implications." *Family Planning Perspectives* 17:53–63.

——— (1986). *Teenage Pregnancy in Industrialized Countries.* New Haven, CT: Yale University Press.

Juster, S. M. (1988). "Disorderly Women: The Feminization of Sin in New England, 1770–1830." Paper presented at the Social Science History Association Meeting, Chicago, October.

Juster, S. M., and M. A. Vinovskis (1987). "Changing Perspectives on the American Family in the Past." *Annual Review of Sociology* 13:193–216.

Kaestle, C. F., and M. A. Vinovskis (1980). *Education and Social Change in Nineteenth-Century Massachusetts.* Cambridge: Cambridge University Press.

Kahn, A. J., and S. B. Kamerman (Eds.) (1988). *Child Support: From Debt Collection to Social Policy.* Newbury Park, CA: Sage.

Kasarda, J. (1985). "Urban Change and Minority Opportunities." In R. E. Peterson (Ed.), *The New Urban Reality.* Washington, DC: Brookings Institution.

Kasun, J. R. (1980). "Adolescent Pregnancy in the United States: An Evaluation of Recent Federal Action." In S. J. Bahr (Ed.), *Economics of the Family.* Lexington, MA: Lexington Books.

Katchadourian, H. (1990). "Sexuality." In S. S. Feldman and G. R. Elliott (Eds.), *At the Threshold: The Developing Adolescent.* Cambridge, MA: Harvard University Press.

Kaus, M. (1986). "The Work Ethic State: The Only Way to Cure the Culture of Poverty." *New Republic* 195, (July):22–33.

Kellam, S. G., R. G. Adams, C. Hendricks Brown, and M. Ensminger (1982). "The Long Term Evolution of the Family Structure of Teenage and Older Mothers." *Journal of Marriage and the Family* 44:539–554.

Keniston, K. (1965). *The Uncommitted: Alienated Youth in American Society.* New York: Harcourt, Brace & World.

Kenney, A. M., J. D. Forrest, and A. Torres (1982). "Storm over Washington: The Parental Notification Proposal." *Family Planning Perspectives* 14: 185–196.

Kessler-Harris, A. (1982). *Out of Work: A History of Wage-earning Women in the U.S.* New York: Oxford University Press.

Kett, J. F. (1977). *Rites of Passage: Adolescence in America, 1790 to the Present.* New York: Basic Books.

Kingdon, John W. (1984). *Agendas, Alternatives, and Public Policies.* Boston: Little, Brown.

Kirby, D. (1983). "The Mathtech Research on Adolescent Sexuality Programs." *SIECUS Report* 12:11–22.

——— (1984). "A Summary of the National Study of Selected Sexuality Programs." *Family Life Educator* 2:24–26.

——— (1985). "Sexuality Education: A More Realistic View of Its Effects." *Journal of School Health* 55:421–424.

——— (1991). "School-based Clinics: Research Results and Their Implications for Future Research Methods." *Evaluation and Program Planning* 14:35–47.

Kirby, D., J. Alter, and P. Scales (1979). *An Analysis of U.S. Sex Education Programs and Evaluation Methods.* Bethesda, MD: Mathtech.

Klerman, L. V. (1975). "Adolescent Pregnancy: The Need for New Policies and New Programs." *Journal of School Health* 45:263–267.

Klerman, L. V., and J. F. Jeckel (1973). *School-Age Mothers: Problems, Programs, and Policy.* Hamden, CT: Linnet.
Kohrman, A. (1988). "Teenage Parenthood: New Directions for Policy in the 1990s." Paper presented at the Public World of Childhood Conference, Chicago, IL, December 2.
Kriesberg, L. (1970). *Mothers in Poverty: A Study of Fatherless Families.* Chicago: Aldine.
Krisberg, B., I. Schwartz, G. Fishman, Z. Eiskovits, and E. Guttman (1986). *The Incarceration of Minority Youth.* Minneapolis: H. H. Humphrey Institute of Public Affairs, University of Minnesota.

Ladner, J. (1971). *Tomorrow's Tomorrow: The Black Woman.* Garden City, NY: Doubleday.
Lancaster, J. B., J. Altmann, A. S. Rossi, and L. R. Sherrod (1987). *Parenting across the Life-Span: Biosocial Dimensions.* New York: Aldine de Gruyter.
Lancaster, J. B., and B. A. Hamburg (1986). "The Biosocial Dimensions of School-Age Pregnancy and Parenthood: An Introduction." In J. Lancaster and B. Hamburg (Eds.), *School-Age Pregnancy and Parenthood: Biosocial Dimensions.* New York: Aldine de Gruyter.
Larson, T. E. (1988). "Employment and Unemployment of Young Black Males." In J. T. Gibbs (Ed.), *Young, Black and Male in America: An Endangered Species.* Dover, MA: Auburn House.
Laslett, P., K. Oosterveen, and R. M. Smith (Eds.) (1980). *Bastardy and Its Comparative History.* Cambridge, MA: Harvard University Press.
Layard, R., and J. Mincer (Eds.) (1985). "Trends in Women's Work, Education, and Family Building. Proceedings of the Conference, Chelwood Gates, Sussex, England, May 31–June 3, 1983." *Journal of Labor Economics* 3, Part 2, S1–S396.
Leacock, E. B. (Ed.) (1971). *The Culture of Poverty: A Critique.* New York: Simon and Schuster.
Lemann, N. (1986). "The Origins of the Underclass." *Atlantic* 258:31–55; 259:54–68.
——— (1991). *The Promised Land: The Great Black Migration and How It Changed America.* New York: Alfred A. Knopf.
Levinson, R. A. (1984). "Contraceptive Self-Efficacy: Primary Prevention." *Journal of Social Work and Human Sexuality* 3:1–15.
——— (1986). "Contraceptive Self-Efficacy: A Perspective on Teenage Girls' Contraceptive Behavior." *Journal of Sex Research* 22:347–369.
Levitan, S. A. (1988). *What's Happening to the American Family? Tensions, Hopes, Realities,* rev. ed. Baltimore: Johns Hopkins Press.
Lewis, O. (1959). *Five Families: Mexican Case Studies in the Culture of Poverty.* New York: Basic Books.
——— (1961). *The Children of Sanchez.* New York: Random House.
——— (1966a). "The Culture of Poverty." *Scientific American* 215:19–25.
——— (1966b). *La Vida: A Puerto Rican Family in the Culture of Poverty—San Juan and New York.* New York: Random House.
Lieberson, S. (1980). *A Piece of the Pie: Black and White Immigrants since 1880.* Berkeley: University of California Press.
Litwack, L. F. (1979). *Been in the Storm So Long: The Aftermath of Slavery.* New York: Knopf.

Lockridge, K. A. (1970). *A New England Town, The First Hundred Years: Dedham, Massachusetts, 1636–1736.* New York: Norton.

Lowi, Theodore P. (1967). "Making Democracy Safe for the World." In J. N. Rosenau (Ed.), *Domestic Sources of Foreign Policy.* New York: Free Press.

Luker, K. (1991). "Dubious Conceptions: The Controversy over Teen Pregnancy." *The American Prospect* 2:73–83.

Lundberg, S., and R. D. Plotnick (1989). "Measuring the Earnings Losses Caused by Teenage Out-of-Wedlock Childbearing." Unpublished paper, University of Washington, Seattle, March.

Lyberg, I. (1984). "Att fråga om barn: Teknisk beskrivning av undersökningen 'Kvinnor och barn.' " Statistics Sweden: Bakgrundsmateriel från Prognosinstitutet, 1984:4.

Lynn, L. E., Jr. (1986). "Public Executives as Policy Makers: Observations on Theory and Practice." Paper presented at the Deuxième Colloque International de la Revue Politiques and Management Public, Lyon.

——— (Ed.). (1989). "Symposium: The Craft of Public Management." *Journal of Policy Analysis and Management* 8:284–306.

McClain, C. (1983). "Criminal Law Reform: Historical Development in the United States." In S. H. Kadish (Ed.), *Encyclopedia of Crime and Justice,* vol. 2. New York: Free Press.

Maccoby, E. E., and C. J. Jacklin (1974). *The Psychology of Sex Differences.* Stanford, CA: Stanford University Press.

McEaddy, B. J. (1976). "Women Who Head Families: A Socio-Economic Analysis." *Monthly Labor Review* 99:3–9.

McLanahan, S. (1986). "Family Structure and Dependency: Early Transitions to Female Household Headships." Institute for Research on Poverty Paper No. 807-86. Madison: University of Wisconsin.

McLanahan, S., and L. Bumpass (1986). "Intergenerational Consequences of Family Disruption." Institute for Research on Poverty Discussion Paper. Madison: University of Wisconsin.

McLanahan, S., and I. Garfinkel (1989). "Single Mothers, the Underclass, and Social Policy." *Annals of the American Academy of Political and Social Science* 501:92–104.

Magnusson, D., H. Stattin, and V. L. Allen (1985). "Biological Maturation and Social Development: A Longitudinal Study of Some Adjustment Processes From Mid-Adolescence to Adulthood." *Journal of Youth and Adolescence* 14:267–283.

Marini, M. M. (1984). "The Transition to Adulthood: Sex Differences in Educational Attainment and Age at Marriage." *American Sociological Review* 49:483–511.

Marsh, J. C. (Ed.) (1991). "Special Issue: Services to Teenage Parents." *Evaluation and Program Planning* 14.

Marshall, W. A., and J. M. Tanner (1969). "Variations in the Pattern of Pubertal Changes in Boys." *Archives of Disease in Childhood* 44:291–303.

——— (1970). "Variations in the Pattern of Pubertal Changes in Girls." *Archives of Disease in Childhood* 45:13–23.

Marsiglio, W. (1987). "Adolescent Fathers in the United States: Their Initial Living Arrangements, Marital Experience, and Educational Outcomes." *Family Planning Perspectives* 11–12:240–251.

Mason, K., M. A. Vinovskis, and T. K. Hareven (1978). "Women's Work and the Life Course in Essex County, Massachusetts, 1880." In T. K. Hareven (Ed.), *Transitions: The Family and the Life Course in Historical Perspective.* New York: Academic Press.

Massachusetts (1887). *Census of Massachusetts, 1885.* 4 vols. Boston: Wright & Potter.

Maxfield, M., Jr. (1990). *Planning Employment Services for the Disadvantaged.* New York: Rockefeller Foundation.

Mead, L. M. (1986). *Beyond Entitlement: The Social Obligations of Citizenship.* New York: Free Press.

Miller, B. C., and K. R. Sneesby (1988). "Educational Correlates of Adolescent Sexual Attitudes and Behavior." *Journal of Youth and Adolescence* 17:521–530.

Miller, S. H. (1983). *Children as Parents.* New York: Child Welfare League of America.

Millman, S. R., and G. E. Hendershot (1980). "Early Fertility and Lifetime Fertility." *Family Planning Perspectives* 12:139–149.

Ministry of Health and Social Affairs (1987). *Yearbook of Health and Social Statistics,* 56. Seoul, Republic of Korea.

Mintz, S., and S. Kellogg (1988). *Domestic Revolutions: A Social History of American Family Life.* New York: Free Press.

Modell, J., and M. Goodman (1990). "Historical Perspectives." In S. S. Feldman and G. R. Elliott (Eds.), *At the Threshold: The Developing Adolescent.* Cambridge, MA: Harvard University Press.

Moore, K. A. (1990). *Facts at a Glance.* Washington, D.C.: Child Trends.

Moore, K. A., and M. R. Burt (1982). *Private Crisis, Public Cost: Policy Perspectives on Teenage Childbearing.* Washington, D.C.: Urban Institute.

Moore, K. A., C. W. Nord, and J. L. Peterson (1989). "Nonvoluntary Sexuality among Adolescents." *Family Planning Perspectives* 21:110–114.

Moore, K. A., and R. F. Werthheimer (1984). "Teenage Childbearing and Welfare: Preventive and Ameliorative Strategies." *Family Planning Perspectives* 16:285–291.

Morgan, E. S. (1966). *The Puritan Family: Religion and Domestic Relations in Seventeenth-Century New England.* New York: Harper & Row.

Morris, N. M., K. Mallin, and J. R. Udry (1982). "Pubertal Development and Current Sexual Intercourse among Teenagers." Paper presented in part at the Annual Meeting of the American Public Health Association, Montreal, November 17.

Mosher, W. D. (1990). "Contraceptive Practice in the United States, 1982–1988." *Family Planning Perspectives* 22:198–205.

Moskos, C. C. (1988). *A Call to Civic Service: National Service for Country and Community.* New York: Free Press.

Moynihan, D. P. (1965). *The Negro Family: The Case For National Action.* Washington: U.S. Department of Labor.

———. (1968). *On Understanding Poverty: Perspectives from the Social Sciences.* New York: Basic Books.

Murray, C. (1984). *Losing Ground: American Social Policy 1950–1980.* New York: Basic Books.

Myrdal, G. (1944). *An American Dilemma: The Negro Problem and Modern Democracy.* New York: Harper & Row.

National Bureau of Statistics (1986). *Korean Statistical Yearbook,* 58. Seoul, Republic of Korea: Economic Planning Board.

National Center for Health Statistics (1962). *Vital Statistics of the United States.* Vol. 1, *Natality.* Washington: GPO.

—— (1984). "Advance Report of Final Natality Statistics, 1982." *Monthly Vital Statistics Report* 33(6):1–44.

—— (1989). "Advance Report of Natality Statistics, 1987." *Monthly Vital Statistics Report* 38(3):1–48.

—— (1990). "Advance Report of Final Natality Statistics, 1988." *Monthly Vital Statistics Report* 39(4):1–48.

—— (1991). "Advance Report of Final Natality Statistics, 1989." *Monthly Vital Statistics Report* 40 (8): 1–56.

National Institute of Drug Abuse (1979). National Survey on Drug Abuse, 1979. Washington: NIDA.

Neimark, E. D. (1975). "Longitudinal Development of Formal Operational Thought." *Genetic Psychology Monographs* 91:171–225.

Nelson, Barbara (1984). *Making an Issue of Child Abuse.* Chicago: University of Chicago Press.

Neugarten, B. L. (1979). "Time, Age and the Life Cycle." *American Journal of Psychiatry* 135:887–894.

Neugarten, B. L., J. W. Moore, and J. C. Lowe (1965). "Age Norms, Age Constraints, and Adult Socialization." *American Journal of Sociology* 70:710–717.

New York State Department of Health (1989). *Birth Outcomes: New York State 1988.* Albany: Office of Public Health Management Group.

New York State Task Force on Poverty and Welfare (1986). *A New Social Contract: Rethinking the Nature and Purpose of Public Assistance.* Report submitted to Governor Mario Cuomo, December.

Newcomer, S. F., and J. R. Udry (1984). "Mothers' Influence on the Sexual Behavior of Their Teenage Children." *Journal of Marriage and the Family* 46:477–485.

Nielsen, J. M., and R. Endo (1983). "Marital Status and Socioeconomic Status: The Case of Female-headed Families." *International Journal of Women Studies* 6:130–147.

Niemi, R. G., J. Mueller, and T. W. Smith (1988). *Trends in Public Opinion: A Compendium of Survey Data.* New York: Greenwood Press.

Nordenstam, U. (1984). "Ha barn—men hur många?" Statistics Sweden: Information i prognosfrågor, 4.

Norton, A. J., and J. E. Moorman (1987). "Current Trends in Marriage and Divorce among American Women." *Journal of Marriage and the Family* 49:3–14.

Novak, M., et al. (1987). *The New Consensus on Family and Welfare: A Community of Self-Reliance.* Washington, D.C.: American Enterprise Institute; Milwaukee: Marquette University Press.

O'Connell, M., and C. C. Rogers (1984). "Out-of-Wedlock Births, Premarital Pregnancies and Their Effect on Family Formation and Dissolution." *Family Planning Perspectives* 16:157–162.

Olson, M. (1965). *The Logic of Collective Action.* Cambridge, MA: Harvard University Press.

Osofsky, J. D., and H. S. Osofsky (1978). "Teenage Pregnancy: Psychological Considerations." *Clinical Obstetrics and Gynecology* 21:1161–1173.

Parker, A. L. (1989). "CBC Legislative Update." *Point of View* (Fall): 83–89.
Pateman, C. (1970). *Participation and Democratic Theory.* Cambridge: Cambridge University Press.
Patterson, J. T. (1986). *America's Struggle against Poverty: 1900–1985.* Cambridge, MA: Harvard University Press.
Petersen, A. C. (1979). "Female Pubertal Development." In M. Sugar (Ed.), *Female Adolescent Development.* New York: Brunner/Mazel.
——— (1980). "Biopsychosocial Processes in the Development of Sex-related Differences." In J. E. Parsons (Ed.), *The Psychology of Sex Differences and Sex Roles.* Washington, DC: Hemisphere.
——— (1983). "Menarche: Meaning of Measures and Measuring Meaning." In S. Golub (Ed.), *Menarche.* New York: Heath.
Petersen, A. C., and A. Boxer (1982). "Adolescent Sexuality." In T. J. Coates, A. C. Petersen, and C. Perry (Eds.), *Promoting Adolescent Health: A Dialog on Research and Practice.* New York: Academic Press.
Petersen, A. C., and L. Crockett (1986). "Pubertal Development and Its Relation to Cognitive and Psychosocial Development in Adolescent Girls: Implications for Parenting." In J. B. Lancaster and B. A. Hamburg (Eds.), *School-Age Pregnancy and Parenthood: Biosocial Dimensions.* New York: Aldine de Gruyter.
Petersen, A. C., A. C. Crouter, and J. Wilson (1988). "Heterosocial Behavior and Sexuality among Normal Young Adolescents." In M. D. Levine and E. R. McAnarney (Eds.), *Early Adolescent Transitions.* Lexington, MA and Toronto: Heath, Lexington Books.
Petersen, A. C., and B. Taylor (1980). "The Biological Approach to Adolescence." In J. Adelson (Ed.), *Handbook of Adolescent Psychology.* New York: Wiley.
Piven, F. (1974). "The Urban Crisis: Who Got What, and Why." In F. Piven and R. Cloward (Eds.), *The Politics of Turmoil.* New York: Pantheon.
Piven, F. F., and R. A. Cloward (1971). *Regulating the Poor: The Functions of Public Welfare.* New York: Pantheon.
Polit, D., and J. Kahn (1985). "Project Redirection: Evaluation of a Comprehensive Program for Disadvantaged Teenage Mothers." *Family Planning Perspectives* 17:150–155.
Polit, D., J. Kahn, and D. Stevens (1985). *Final Impacts from Project Redirection.* New York: Manpower Development Research Center.
Polsky, A. J. (1991). *The Rise of the Therapeutic State.* Princeton, NJ: Princeton University Press.
Popenoe, D. (1987). "Beyond Tradition: A Statistical Portrait of the Changing Family in Sweden." *Journal of Marriage and the Family* 49:173–183.
President's Science Advisory Committee, Panel on Youth (1974). *Youth: Transition to Adulthood.* Chicago: University of Chicago Press.
Price, D. E. (1978). "Policymaking in Congressional Committees: The Impact of Environmental Factors." *American Political Science Review* 72:161–188.
Putnam, F. W. (1990). "Developmental Antecedents of Dissociative Disorders: Contributions to Criminality?" Presented at Workshop on Gender Issues in the Development of Devious Behavior, Henry A. Murray Research Center, Radcliffe College, Cambridge, MA, June 1990.

Rainwater, L. (1966). "Crucible of Identity: The Negro Lower Class Family." *Daedalus* 95:172–216.

——— (1987). "Class, Culture, Poverty, and Welfare." Unpublished manuscript, Harvard University, Department of Sociology.

Rainwater, L., and L. Yancey (1967). *The Moynihan Report and the Politics of Controversy.* Cambridge, MA: MIT Press.

Rapoport, L. (1962). "The State of Crisis: Some Theoretical Considerations." *Social Service Review* 36:211–217.

Reed, J. (1983). *The Birth Control Movement and American Society: From Private Vice to Public Virtue,* rev. ed. Princeton, NJ: Princeton University Press.

Reed, R. J. (1988). "Education and Achievement of Young Black Males." In J. T. Gibbs (Ed.), *Young, Black and Male in America: An Endangered Species.* Dover, MA: Auburn House.

Rein, M., and H. Heclo (1973). "What Welfare Crisis? A Comparison among the United States, Britain, and Sweden." *Public Interest* 33:61–83.

Ricketts, E. R., and I. V. Sawhill (1986). "Defining and Measuring the Underclass." Paper preseted at the American Economic Association, New Orleans.

Rindfuss, R. R., C. G. Swicegood, and R. A. Rosenfeld (1987). "Disorder in the Life-Course: How Common and Does It Matter?" *American Sociological Review* 52:785–801.

Robbins, C., H. B. Kaplan, and S. S. Martin (1985). "Antecedents of Pregnancy among Unmarried Adolescents." *Journal of Marriage and the Family* 47:567–583.

Robinson, B. (1988). *Teenage Fathers.* Lexington, MA: Lexington Books.

Rodgers, H. R. (1986). *Poor Women, Poor Families: The Economic Plight of America's Female-headed Households.* Armonk, NY: M. E. Sharpe.

Rolén, M., and P. Springfeldt (1987). "Make och far." Statistics Sweden: Demografiska rapporter, 2.

Rosenbaum, J. E., T. Kariya, R. Settersten, and T. Maier (1990). "Market and Network Theories of the Transition from High School to Work: Their Application to Industrialized Societies." *Annual Review of Sociology* 16:263–299.

Rosenheim, M. K. (1966). "Vagrancy Concepts in Welfare Law." In J. tenBroek (Ed.), *The Law of the Poor.* San Francisco: Chandler.

——— (1976). "Notes on Helping Juvenile Nuisances." In M. K. Rosenheim (Ed.), *Pursuing Justice for the Child.* Studies in Crime and Justice. Chicago and London: University of Chicago Press.

Ross, H. L., and I. V. Sawhill (1975). *Time of Transition: The Growth of Families Headed by Women.* Washington, D.C.: Urban Institute.

Russo, A., and L. Humphreys (1983). "Homosexuality and Crime." In S. H. Kadish (Ed.), *Encyclopedia of Crime and Justice,* vol. 2. New York: Free Press.

Sadler, L. S., and C. Catrone (1983). "The Adolescent Parent: A Dual Developmental Crisis." *Journal of Adolescent Health Care* 4:100–105.

Sampson, R. (1992) "Family Management and Child Development: Insights from Social Disorganization Theory." In J. McCord (Ed.), *Advances in Criminological Theory,* vol. 3. New Brunswick, N.J.: Transaction.

Sander, J. H., and J. L. Rosen (1987). "Teenage Fathers: Working With the Neglected Partner in Adolescent Childbearing." *Family Planning Perspectives* 19:107–110.

Sandqvist, K. (1987). "Swedish Family Policy and the Attempt to Change Parental Roles." In C. Lewis and M. O'Brien (Eds.), *Reassessing Fatherhood: New Observations on Fathers and the Modern Family.* London: Sage.

Sarigiani, P. A., J. Wilson, A. C. Petersen, and J. Vicary (1990). "Self-Image and Educational Plans of Adolescents from Two Contrasting Communities." *Journal of Early Adolescence* 10:37–55.

Schattschneider, E. E. (1960). *The Semi-Sovereign People.* New York: Holt, Rinehart & Winston.

Schlossman, S. L. (1977). *Love and the American Delinquent: The Theory and Practice of Progressive Juvenile Justice, 1825–1920.* Chicago: University of Chicago Press.

Schlossman, S., and S. Wallach (1980). "The Crime of Precocious Sexuality: Female Juvenile Delinquency in the Progressive Era." *Harvard Educational Review* 48:65–94.

Schorr, A. (1986). *Common Decency: Domestic Politics after Reagan.* New Haven, CT: Yale University Press.

Schorr, L. B. (1988). *Within Our Reach: Breaking the Cycle of Disadvantage.* Garden City, NY: Doubleday.

Schulz, D. A. (1969). *Coming Up Black: Patterns of Ghetto Socialization.* Englewood Cliffs, NJ: Prentice-Hall.

Schur, E. M. (1988). *The Americanization of Sex.* Philadelphia: Temple University Press.

Schwartz, S. (1973). "Effects of Sex Guilt and Sexual Arousal on the Retention of Birth Control Information." *Journal of Consulting and Clinical Psychology* 44:61–64.

Sherraden, M. W., and D. J. Eberly (Eds.) (1982). *National Service: Social, Economic and Military Impacts.* New York: Pergamon.

Shinn, M. (1978). "Father Absence and Children's Cognitive Development." *Psychological Bulletin* 85:295–324.

Siegel, E., and N. M. Morris (1974). "Family Planning: Its Health Rationale." *American Journal of Obstetrics and Gynecology* 118:995–1003.

Siim, B. (1987). "The Scandinavian Welfare States—Towards Sexual Equality or a New Kind of Male Domination?" *Acta Sociologica* 30:255–270.

Simmons, R. G., and D. A. Blyth (1987). *Moving into Adolescence: The Impact of Pubertal Change and School Context.* Hawthorne, NY: Aldine.

Singh, S. (1986). "Adolescent Pregnancy in the United States: An Interstate Analysis." *Family Planning Perspectives* 9–10:210–220.

Slovenko, R. (1983). "Adultery and Fornication." In S. H. Kadish (Ed.), *Encyclopedia of Crime and Justice,* vol. 1. New York: Free Press.

Stack, C. (1974). *All Our Kin.* New York: Harper & Row.

Starr, P., and E. Immergut (1987). "Health Care and the Boundaries of Politics." In C. Maier (Ed.), *Changing Boundaries of the Political: Essays on the Evolving Balance between State and Society, Public and Private in Europe.* Cambridge: Cambridge University Press.

Steiner, G. Y. (1971). *The State of Welfare.* Washington, D.C.: Brookings Institution.

Stiles, H. R. (1934). *Bundling: Its Origin, Progress, and Decline in America.* New York: Book Collectors Association.

Stone, D. (1989). "Causal Stories and the Formation of Policy Agendas." *Political Science Quarterly* 104:281–300.

Stout, J. W., and F. P. Rivara (1989). "Schools and Sex Education: Does It Work?" *Pediatrics* 83:375–379.

Sullivan, M. (1986). "Ethnographic Research on Young Fathers and Parenting: Implications for Public Policy." Paper prepared for the Young Unwed Fatherhood Symposium, Catholic University, Washington, DC, October. SHARE, Bethesda, MD. SHR-0015257.

Sum, A., P. Harrington, and W. Goedicke (1987). "One-Fifth of the Nation's Teenagers: Employment Problems of Poor Youth in America, 1981–1985." *Youth and Society* 18:195–237.

Sundstrom, M. (1987). "A Study in the Growth of Part-Time Work in Sweden." Stockholm: Arbetslivscentrum and Almqvist & Wiksell International.

Sung, K. (1985). "A Study of Issues regarding Unwed Mothers, Child Abandonment, and Adoption." Report prepared for Terre Des Hommes, West Germany.

――― (1987). "Koreans' Attitudes toward the Family." Paper presented to the Center for East Asian Studies, University of Chicaago, February 1989.

―――. (1990). "A New Look at Filial Piety: Ideals and Practices of Family-Centered Care in Korea." *The Gerontologist* 30:610–617.

Susman, E. J., G. Inoff-Germain, E. D. Nottelmann, D. L. Loriaux, G. B. Cutler, Jr., and G. P. Chrousos (1987). "Hormones, Emotional Dispositions, and Aggressive Attributes in Young Adolescents." *Child Development* 58: 1114–1134.

Tanner, J. M. (1972). "Sequence, Tempo, and Individual Variation in Growth and Development of Boys and Girls Aged Twelve to Sixteen." In J. Kagan and R. Coles (Eds.), *Twelve to Sixteen: Early Adolescence.* New York: Norton.

Teitelbaum, L. E., and A. R. Gough (Eds.). (1977). *Beyond Control: Status Offenders in the Juvenile Court.* Cambridge, MA: Ballinger.

Teitelbaum, L. E., and L. J. Harris (1977). "Some Historical Perspectives on Governmental Regulation of Children and Parents." In L. E. Teitelbaum and A. R. Gough (Eds.), *Beyond Control: Status Offenders in the Juvenile Court.* Cambridge, MA: Ballinger.

Testa, M., N. M. Astone, M. Krogh, and K. M. Neckerman (1989). "Employment and Marriage among Inner-City Fathers." *Annals of the American Academy of Political and Social Sciences* 501:79–91.

Testa, M., and M. Krogh (1990). "Nonmarital Parenthood, Male Joblessness and AFDC Participation in Inner-City Chicago: Final Report." Prepared for Office of the Assistant Secretary for Planning and Evaluation, U.S. Department of Health and Human Services, Grant 88ASPE204A.

Testa, M., and E. Lawlor (1985). *The State of the Child.* Chicago: Chapin Hall Center, University of Chicago.

Thompson, K. (1980). "A Comparison of Black and White Adolescents' Beliefs about Having Children." *Journal of Marriage and the Family* 42:133–139.

Thompson, R. (1986). *Sex in Middlesex: Popular Mores in a Massachusetts County, 1649–1699.* Amherst: University of Massachusetts Press.

Tobin-Richards, M. H., A. M. Boxer, and A. C. Petersen (1983). "The Psychological Significance of Pubertal Change." In J. Brooks-Gunn and A. C. Petersen (Eds.), *Girls at Puberty: Biological and Psychosocial Perspectives.* New York: Plenum.

Torres, A., and J. D. Forrest (1985). "Family Planning Clinic Services in the United States." *Family Planning Perspectives* 17:30–35.

Tracy, P. J. (1979). *Jonathan Edwards, Pastor: Religion and Society in Eighteenth-Century Northampton.* New York: Hill & Wang.

Tribe, L. (1990). *Abortion: The Clash of Absolutes.* New York: Norton.

Trickett, P. K., and F. W. Putnam (1987). "The Psychobiological Effects of Sexual Abuse: Female Growth and Development during Childhood and Adolescence." Grant funded by W.T. Grant Foundation. Chesapeake Institute, Wheaton, MD.

Trickett, P. K., F. W. Putnam, and R. J. Weinstein (1990). "Timing of Maturation and Negative Affect and Behavior in Sexually Abused Girls." Presentation in the symposium "Biological, Familial, and Psychological Influences on the Development of Depressive Affect and Behavior in Adolescence" at the Biennial Meeting of the Society for Research on Adolescence, Atlanta, March.

Trilling, L. (1953). *The Liberal Imagination.* Garden City, NY: Doubleday.

Troll, L. E., and V. Bengtson (1982). "Intergenerational Relations throughout the Life Span." In B. Wolman (Ed.), *Handbook of Developmental Psychology.* Englewood Cliffs, NJ: Prentice-Hall.

Trost, J., and B. Lewin (1978). Att sambo och gifta sig: Fakta och föreställningar. Stockholm: Statens offentliga utredningar, 55.

Udry, J. R. (1982). "Socialization of Adolescent Sexual Behavior: A Comparison of Findings for Blacks and Whites." Presented at the Annual Meeting of the National Council on Family Relations, Washington, D.C., October.

Udry, J. R., and J. O. Billy (1987). "Initiation of Coitus in Early Adolescence." *American Sociological Review* 52:841–855.

Udry, J. R., J. O. Billy, N. M. Morris, T. R. Groff, and M. H. Raj (1985). "Serum Androgenic Hormones Motivate Sexual Behavior in Adolescent Boys." *Sterility and Fertility* 43:90–94.

Udry, J. R., L. M. Talbert, and N. M. Morris (1986). "Biosocial Foundations for Adolescent Female Sexuality." *Demography* 23:217–230.

Upchurch, D. M., and J. McCarthy (1990). "The Timing of a First Birth and High School Completion." *American Sociological Review* 55:224–234.

U.S. Bureau of the Census (1953). *U.S. Census of the Population: 1950.* Vol. II, *Characteristics of the Population,* part I, United States Summary. Washington: GPO.

——— (1987a). *Current Population Reports.* Series P-60, No. 157. "Money Income and Poverty Status of Families and Persons in the United States: 1986." Washington: GPO.

——— (1987b). *Statistical Abstract of the United States, 1987,* 107th ed. Washington: GPO.

——— (1990). *Marital Status and Living Arrangements: March 1989.* Current Population Reports, Series P-20, No. 445. Washington: GPO.

——— (1991a). *School Enrollment—Social and Economic Characteristics of Students: October 1989.* Current Population Reports, Series P-20, No. 452. Washington: GPO.

—— (1991*b*). *Marital Status and Living Arrangements: March 1990.* Current Population Reports, Series P-20, No. 450. Washington: GPO.

U.S. Commission on Civil Rights (1983). "A Growing Crisis: Disadvantaged Women and Their Children." Clearinghouse Publication 78. Washington: GPO.

U.S. Congress, House, Select Committee on Population (1978). "Fertility and Contraception in the United States." 95th Cong., 2d Sess., Serial B.

U.S. Department of Health and Human Services (1986). *Report of the Secretary's Task Force on Black and Minority Health,* vol. 5. Washington: DHHS.

Valentine, C. A. (1968). *Culture and Poverty: Critique and Counter Proposals.* Chicago: University of Chicago Press.

Vance, C. (1984). *Pleasure and Danger.* London: Routledge & Kegan Paul.

Vicary, J. R. (1985). "Psychological Impact of Pregnancy for Rural Adolescent Girls." PHS grant APR 000933-03. Department of Human Development and Family Studies, College of Health and Human Development, Pennsylvania State University, xerox.

Vinovskis, M. A. (1981). *Fertility in Massachusetts from the Revolution to the Civil War.* New York: Academic Press.

—— (1986*a*). "Adolescent Sexuality and Childbearing in Early America." In J. B. Lancaster and B. A. Hamburg (Eds.), *School-Age Pregnancy and Parenthood: Biosocial Dimensions.* New York: Aldine de Gruyter.

—— (1986*b*). "Young Fathers and Their Children: Some Historical and Policy Perspectives." In A. B. Elster and M. E. Lamb (Eds.), *Adolescent Fatherhood.* Hillsdale, NJ: L. Erlbaum.

—— (1988*a*). *An "Epidemic" of Adolescent Pregnancy? Some Historical and Policy Perspectives.* New York: Oxford University Press.

—— (1988*b*). "Teenage Pregnancy and the Underclass." *Public Interest* 93: 87–96.

—— (1988*c*). "The Unravelling of the Family Wage since World War II: Some Demographic, Economic, and Cultural Considerations." In B. Christensen (Ed.), *The Family Wage: Work, Gender, and Children in the Modern Economy.* Rockford, IL: Rockford Institute.

Vinovskis, M. A., and P. L. Chase-Lansdale (1988). "Hasty Marriages or Hasty Conclusions?" *Public Interest* 90:128–132.

Vogel, J. (1986). Sysselsättningskrisen påverkar ungdomarnas familjebildning. Statistics Sweden: *Välfärdsbulletinen,* 1:3.

Voydanoff, P., and B. W. Donnelly (1990). *Adolescent Sexuality and Pregnancy.* Newbury Park, CA: Sage.

Walker, J. L. (1977). "Setting the Agenda in the U.S. Senate: A Theory of Problem Selection." *British Journal of Political Science* 7:412–445.

Weatherley, R. A., S. B. Perlman, M. H. Levine, and L. V. Klerman (1986). "Comprehensive Programs for Pregnant Teenagers and Teenage Parents: How Successful Have They Been?" *Family Planning Perspectives* 18:73–78.

Weeks, J. R. (1976). *Teenage Marriages: A Demographic Analysis.* Westport, CT: Greenwood Press.

Weitzman, L. J. (1985). *The Divorce Revolution: The Unexpected Social and Economic Consequences for Women and Children in America.* New York: Free Press.

Wells, R. V. (1985). *Uncle Sam's Family: Issues in and Perspectives on American Demographic History.* Albany: State University of New York Press.

Werner, E. E., and R. S. Smith (1982). *Vulnerable But Invincible.* New York: McGraw-Hill.

Wikman, R. (1937). "Die Einleitung der Ehe. Eine vergleichend ethnosoziologische Untersuchung uber die Vorstufe der Ehe in den Sitten des schwedishen Volkstums." *Acta Academiae Abonensis, Humaniora XI,* 1, 1–395. Turku: Åbo Akademi.

Williams, J. (Ed.) (1982). *The State of Black America, 1982.* New York: National Urban League.

Williams, T., and W. Kornblum (1985). *Growing Up Poor.* Lexington, MA: Lexington Books.

W. T. Grant Foundation (1988a). *The Forgotten Half: Non-College Youth in America.* Washington, DC: W. T. Grant Foundation Commission on Work, Family and Citizenship.

——— (1988b). *The Forgotten Half: Pathways to Success.* Washington, DC: W. T. Grant Foundation Commission on Work, Family and Citizenship.

Wilson, W. J. (1987). *The Truly Disadvantaged.* Chicago: University of Chicago Press.

——— (Ed.) (1989). "The Ghetto Underclass, Social Science Perspectives." Special issue of *The Annals of the American Academy of Political and Social Science* 501.

Wilson, W. J., and K. M. Neckerman (1984). "Poverty and Family Structure: The Widening Gap between Evidence and Public Policy Issues." Paper prepared for Conference on Poverty and Policy: Retrospect and Prospects. Williamsburg, VA. December 6–8.

——— (1987). "Poverty and Family Structure: The Widening Gap between Evidence and Public Policy Issues." In W. J. Wilson (Ed.), *The Truly Disadvantaged.* Chicago: University of Chicago Press.

Winnicott, D. W. (1971). *Playing and Reality.* New York: Penguin.

Woofter, T. J. (1971 [1920]). *Negro Migration: Changes in Rural Organization and Population of the Cotton Belt.* Reprint. New York: AMS Press.

——— (1930). *Black Yeomanry: Life on St. Helena's Island.* New York: Holt.

World Fertility Survey (1984). *Fertility Survey in Sweden, 1981.* International Statistical Institute, Voorburg, The Netherlands: World Fertility Survey, Summaries of Findings, No. 43.

Wyshak, G., and R. E. Frisch (1982). "Evidence for a Secular Trend in Age of Menarche." *New England Journal of Medicine* 306:245–306.

Zabin, L. S., M. B. Hirsch, E. A. Smith, R. Strett, and J. B. Hardy (1986). "Evaluation of a Pregnancy Prevention Program for Urban Teenagers." *Family Planning Perspectives* 11:215–222.

Zelnik, M., and J. F. Kanter (1980). "Sexual Activity, Contraceptive Use and Pregnancy among Metropolitan Area Teenagers: 1971–1979." *Family Planning Perspectives* 12:230–237.

Zelnik, M., J. F. Kanter, and K. Ford (1983). *Adolescent Pathways to Pregnancy.* Beverly Hills: Sage.

Zimring, F. E. (1982). *The Changing Legal World of Adolescence.* New York: Free Press; London: Collier Macmillan.

Contributors

Andrew Boxer is director of the Center for Gay and Lesbian Mental Health and assistant professor, Department of Psychiatry, the University of Chicago. He has published papers on many facets of adolescence and conducts research on adolescent development, sexuality, and parent-child relations.

Evelyn Brodkin is associate professor, School of Social Service Administration and the College, and teaches as well in the Graduate School of Public Policy and the School of Law, at the University of Chicago. Professor Brodkin writes on social welfare policy, and is the author of *The False Promise of Administrative Reform: Implementing Quality Control in Welfare.*

Jeanne Brooks-Gunn is the Virginia and Leonard Marx Professor in Child and Parent Development and Education and Director, Center for the Development and Education of Young Children and Their Parents at Teachers College, Columbia University. She is also senior research scientist and director of the Adolescent Study Program at the Educational Testing Service. A developmental psychologist, she studies families and children, with a special emphasis on the biological and social factors that render children and youth at risk for school, relational, and emotional problems. Her recent books include *Adolescent Mothers in Later Life,*

The Encyclopedia of Adolescence, and *The Development of Depression during Adolescence.*

Lisa J. Crockett is assistant professor of Human Development at the Pennsylvania State University. Her research examines biological, psychological, and social development in adolescence with a focus on the processes leading to positive and negative adjustment.

Sandra Lee Dixon is a doctoral candidate in Religion and the Human Sciences at the Divinity School, the University of Chicago. Her research interests are moral psychology and the contributions of unconscious and cultural factors to moral thought.

Donna L. Franklin is associate professor at the School of Social Service Administration, the University of Chicago. She is the author of many scholarly articles on topics including the feminization of poverty, adolescent sexuality and fertility, epistemological issues in social work practice, and race and class as they affect social work.

Frank F. Furstenberg, Jr., is professor in the Department of Sociology, University of Pennsylvania, where he also holds appointments in the School of Medicine and the Population Studies Center. Professor Furstenberg's research has addressed family issues, specifically adolescent pregnancy, sexuality and childbearing, and the effect of divorce on the family. His books include *Unplanned Parenthood: The Social Consequences of Teenage Childbearing* and *Adolescent Mothers in Later Life.*

Jewelle Taylor Gibbs is professor in the School of Social Welfare, University of California at Berkeley. Her research has focused on the effects of ethnicity, social class, and gender on the psychosocial adjustment of adolescents. She is the editor of *Young, Black and Male in America: An Endangered Species* and the coauthor of *Children of Color: Psychological Interventions with Minority Youth.*

Beatrix Hamburg is professor of Psychiatry and Pediatrics and director, Division of Child and Adolescent Psychiatry, Mount Sinai School of

Medicine, New York. She is author of many articles on adolescence as well as coeditor of *School-Age Pregnancy and Parenthood: Biosocial Dimensions*. She served on the panel of the National Research Council that produced the study *Risking the Future: Adolescent Sexuality, Pregnancy, and Childbearing*.

Britta Hoem is research associate in the Section of Demography at the University of Stockholm. She was Honorary Visitor in the Center for Demography and Ecology at the University of Wisconsin–Madison in 1988. She has written articles in both Swedish and English on topics including childbearing, cohabitation and marriage, divorce and union dissolution, and population forecasting.

Mary Elizabeth Hughes is a doctoral candidate in sociology and demography at the Population Studies Center, University of Pennsylvania. Her research interest is social demography, specifically fertility and labor force issues concerning women and mature adults.

Anne C. Petersen is Vice President for Research and Dean of the Graduate School at the University of Minnesota. Her books include *Girls at Puberty: Biological and Psychosocial Perspectives,* and her research examines the interactions among cognitive, social, biological, and emotional development from late childhood into early adulthood.

Margaret K. Rosenheim is Helen Ross Professor in the School of Social Service Administration, the University of Chicago. Her interests lie in the history of social welfare, public policy for children, and juvenile justice. She is the editor of *Pursuing Justice for the Child.*

Kyu-taik Sung is professor in the Department of Social Work, Yonsei University, Seoul, Korea. He has written on family planning services in both the United States and Korea, and on programs for teenage mothers in the United States. He is author of *Evaluation of the Organizational Effectiveness of Family Planning Clinics* and *Medical Ethics: The State of Public Health and Medical Care in Korea.*

Mark F. Testa is associate professor at the School of Social Service Administration, the University of Chicago, and faculty associate for the Chapin Hall Center for Children. He coauthored *The State of the Child: 1985* and *The State of the Child* (1980) and is conducting a five-state study, "The Comparative State of the Child."

Maris Vinovskis is professor in the Department of History and research scientist in the Center for Political Studies, Institute for Social Research, at the University of Michigan. He has studied the family, demography, and abortion in American history. The author of *An "Epidemic" of Adolescent Pregnancy? Some Historical and Policy Considerations,* he also served on the panel of the National Research Council that produced *Risking the Future.*

Franklin E. Zimring is professor in the School of Law and director of the Earl Warren Legal Institute, University of California, Berkeley. He is the author of several books and many articles on juvenile justice, domestic relations, and criminal law, including *The Changing Legal World of Adolescence.*

Index

D